Diets Designed for Athletes

Maryann Karinch

Human Kinetics

Library of Congress Cataloging-in-Publication Data

Karinch, Maryann
   Diets designed for athletes / Maryann Karinch.
     p. cm.
   Includes bibliographical references and index.
   ISBN 0-7360-3834-5
    1. Athletes--Nutrition. 2. Diet. I. Title.

   TX361.A8 K37 2001
   613.2'024'796--dc21

                                         2001039409

ISBN: 0-7360-3834-5

Acquisitions Editor: Martin Barnard; **Developmental Editor:** Cassandra Mitchell; **Assistant Editor:** Dan Brachtesende; **Copyeditor:** Karen L. Marker; **Proofreader:** Coree Schutter; **Indexer:** Nancy Ball; **Permission Manager:** Toni Harte; **Graphic Designer:** Nancy Rasmus; **Graphic Artist:** Tara Welsch; **Photo Manager:** Tom Roberts; **Cover Designer:** Keith Blomberg; **Art Managers:** Craig Newsom and Carl Johnson; **Illustrator:** Tom Roberts; **Printer:** Bang Printing

Human Kinetics books are available at special discounts for bulk purchase. Special editions or book excerpts can also be created to specification. For details, contact the Special Sales Manager at Human Kinetics.

Printed in the United States of America   10 9 8 7 6 5 4 3 2 1

Human Kinetics
Web site: www.humankinetics.com

United States: Human Kinetics, P.O. Box 5076, Champaign, IL 61825-5076
800-747-4457
e-mail: humank@hkusa.com

Canada: Human Kinetics, 475 Devonshire Road Unit 100, Windsor, ON N8Y 2L5
800-465-7301 (in Canada only)
e-mail: orders@hkcanada.com

Europe: Human Kinetics, Units C2/C3 Wira Business Park, West Park Ring Road
Leeds LS16 6EB, United Kingdom
+44 (0) 113 278 1708
e-mail: hk@hkeurope.com

Australia: Human Kinetics, 57A Price Avenue, Lower Mitcham, South Australia 5062
08 8277 1555
e-mail: liahka@senet.com.au

New Zealand: Human Kinetics, P.O. Box 105-231, Auckland Central
09-523-3462
e-mail: hkp@ihug.co.nz

To my mother, my brother, Jim, Mary Helen, and Dean—may good meals and love continue to bring us together.

CONTENTS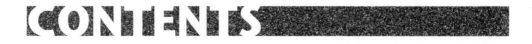

ACKNOWLEDGMENTS

To all of my friends and relatives who sent bars, saved wrappers, faxed articles, and e-mailed me your opinions about products designed for athletes: thank you. As always, Jim McCormick gave generously of his time and intelligence to help me organize my thoughts; he also located places to store my tubs of protein powder, sport drinks, packets of gel, energy snacks, and supplements. Mom's encouragement, thoughtful discussion, and prayers helped a lot, too, as did my brother's steady belief in me and his healthy skepticism about food that comes from labs. I got first-class support, advice, and representation from my agent, Laura Belt, and I feel as though my diligent editor, Cassandra Mitchell, and I forged a true partnership. Thank you both. I also appreciate Martin Barnard's willingness to commit Human Kinetics to this project and Toni Harte's persistence with permissions. The HK team is superb!

As I studied, read, interviewed, tasted, and tested my way through the development of this book, I often had more questions than answers. Thank you heartily to the experts outside and inside the industry who helped me sort through the information. A special acknowledgment goes to David Sherer, MD who reviewed the tough questions from my distinguished expert reviewers and helped me provide clear answers. A practicing anesthesiologist, David is also a competitive runner and co-author with me of an upcoming book on hospital safety for patients. I appreciate that he took time away from his newborn son, Liam, and his "firstborn," a golden retriever named Freddie, to research complicated issues regarding health-related risks and claims and physiological processes. Thank you also to Jay Sanders, MD for his medical insights. And, certainly, this book is so much richer and more useful because of the input from industry pioneers and leaders who explained why and how they developed their products: Mike Carnazzo, Dr. Scott Connelly, Brian Frank, Dr. Doug Herthel, Mark Herthel, Dr. Lee H. Lorenzen, David Jenkins, Brian Maxwell, Jennifer (Biddulph) Maxwell, Dr. Barry Sears,

Jim Valente, Dr. Bill Vaughan, Jim Warren, and Michael Zumpano. Thank you also to the people who do a superior job of communicating the function and value of certain types of products and nutritional approaches to enhancing athletic performance: Dr. Nick Abrishamian, Mike Bottom, Dr. Priscilla M. Clarkson, Chad Coy, Steve Fluet, Rob Fulcomer, Ric Giardina, Dr. Paul Hutinger, Nate Llerandi, Kevin Maselka, Dr. Bill Misner, Alex Rogers, and Greg Zoeller.

   Much of the book's life also comes from the stories and insights of dedicated elite athletes: Tao Berman, Lori Bowden, Tony DeBoom, Will Gadd, Wes Hobson, Linda Holland, Heidi Howkins, Jim McCormick, Mohamad (Moe) Moussawi, Bryan Neese, Michael Powers, Peter Reid, Cathy Sassin, Lisa Smith, and Dara Torres. People who work for companies in the industry and for sports publications and associations did so much to help me locate important research and get in touch with top athletes. I really appreciate the contributions of Cassie Cyphers, Christine Evans, Carl House, Doug Jones, Jack Kavulich, Julie Atherton McFadden, Jason Stephens, Mike Stott, Phil Whitten, and Larry Zoeller. Finally, blasting into the past, I want to thank Tony Wagner, my bodybuilding coach, whose guidance awakened my interest in designing diets for athletes.

INTRODUCTION

Athletes, here are three facts you need to improve your performance with sports foods: (1) every body is different; (2) you need to look at your whole nutritional picture, not just a piece of it; and (3) what you put in your mouth doesn't necessarily get absorbed by your body.

To address the first point, this book gives you information to help you match your unique needs with specially formulated products. You may be a runner or a bodybuilder who wants to reach a higher level, but modeling your diet on the eating habits of your favorite runner or bodybuilder won't necessarily serve you well. A host of factors can make your needs very different from those of another athlete who competes in the same sport: your metabolism, the altitude where you live and train, a medical condition, and more. If you try to use someone else's formula, you may see some changes—maybe a little more energy, for example—but then again, the new regimen might make no difference at all to your performance. Or your energy might actually decrease.

An elite athlete's diet may be a good starting point, but to make the proper adjustment you need to pay attention to how you feel before, during, and after each workout. The world's best athletes don't eat the same way or use the same products—even those in the same sport—because they have learned over time what works precisely right for them.

A couple of days after I wrote the section on sports drinks for use during and after endurance activities, I talked with Lisa Smith, a top ultra-runner and multisport adventure racer. She is one of several elite endurance athletes who rely on protein drinks as much as carbohydrate drinks during events. Considering that her events often exceed 24 hours, that didn't seem so odd; it was what she told me afterward that sent me racing to add new material to this introduction. Lisa mentioned a fellow ultra-runner who routinely powers through races of 100 miles or more by downing a Coca-Cola every 10 miles. "That's an intriguing footnote to my research," I thought. I had just written my caution to athletes about avoiding carbonated, caffeinated, sugary beverages during and after races because they cause bloating, excessive urination, and uneven energy—for most people in the studies. The man who runs on cola is obviously not like "most people in the studies". What I've tried to do in this book is tell you what should work best in different circumstances, what athletes who have tried different products believe works for them, and what manufacturers of performance-enhancing products intend that their products do for you. But no matter what insights you use as your starting point, you will still need to go through a process of refining your food and supplement choices according to how you feel.

The second point—that you must look at the whole picture—came out of a conversation with Steve Fluet, who is both an athlete and a trainer. We went back and forth about the value of different products and the challenge of recommending when and how often to ingest them. You have to look at these bars, drinks, and gels in the context of your whole training and nutrition program. You don't want to find yourself ruled by the promises associated with them, such as, "One of these will give you hours of energy." Sure, you can flip to the energy bar chart to figure out what to buy today because you only have a 30-minute window to eat before your workout. It's better than guessing. But that approach doesn't support a program of performance improvement; it doesn't take into consideration the other foods you eat, your training schedule, and the fact that you have a race in two weeks.

When you use performance-enhancing products, you want the results to be predictable—and the only way to get predictable results is to fit the products you use into the big picture of training, eating, and competing. If you bonk one day during a workout, you can get yourself back on track by answering questions like these:

What did I eat and drink yesterday? Today?

How much sleep did I get last night?

When was the last time I bonked?

What did I eat the day before that happened? The day it happened?

What did I eat after I bonked? How did that make me feel?

When was the last time I had a great workout?

What was different about what I ate beforehand, or how much I slept?

Were there any differences in health, climate, stress level, or other factors that can affect digestion, the requirement for certain nutrients, and performance?

Finally, if you know that your body doesn't absorb everything you put in your mouth, you can start to fine-tune your diet to an even greater degree. Whether or not you get the intended benefits of foods you eat depends on a lot of factors, such as the quality of the product and your timing in ingesting them. This book will help you to choose wisely based on your performance targets and requirements, to determine appropriate portions and dosages, and to set up a schedule to maximize benefits of the whole foods and products.

Let this book help you make good investments in products, understand your reactions to them, and discover when and how to make adjustments to improve your athletic performance. Use the information to decide how to fit nutrition products into your overall program. Resist the urge to address individual athletic problems or challenges with a series of quick fixes that may not make sense together.

When you integrate products that make sense for you into a diet that supports your athletic goals, you'll feel the difference quickly and other athletes will see it. People will start asking, "What's your secret?" Let me know when that happens so I can tell your story, too.

CHAPTER 1

Using Performance-Enhancing Foods

In the 24th-century world of *Star Trek*, computers produce perfect food instantly. Before you can utter "nonmeat protein dish rich in folic acid," *voilà*, a bowl of steaming yellow pea-and-spinach soup appears. It's not quite that easy in the 21st century, but engineered foods do aim to combine good nutrition with convenience.

In most cases, these bars, gels, drinks, capsules, and powders are formulated to be much more than a convenient food source for athletes. They target the energy, recovery, and body composition needs associated with a particular sport or physical regimen. They help you maintain lean body mass while providing the chemical components your body needs to maintain an optimum balance. In conjunction with a "real food" diet that focuses similarly on performance gains and advantages, these products can serve you well.

You might wonder why you would need specially formulated foods and supplements if you pay close attention to your diet and follow guidelines such as the United States government's Dietary Reference Intakes (DRIs), the latest revision of the Recommended Dietary Allowances (RDAs). The nutrient levels suggested by the DRIs for a high-performance athlete may actually be difficult or impossible to meet by eating whole foods alone. The nutrition scientists on the Food and Nutrition Board of the National Academy of Sciences who generated the DRIs, therefore, acknowledge the value of supplementation in many diets. As a devoted athlete, you subject yourself to unusual environmental stresses—you work at a different rate from the general population—and that can dramatically raise your macronutrient and micronutrient requirements.

Hard training creates measurable deficiencies that can result in a range of physical problems. Many studies have looked at what nutrients athletes lose through hard training and concluded that athletes often need supplements to stay healthy. In the push to be stronger, go longer, or reshape your body you sweat out electrolytes such as magnesium, potassium, and sodium. You place added demands on free radical scavengers such as vitamin E. Intense training also lowers glutamine levels and that can jeopardize your immune system.

One study that focused on trace elements was conducted by the U.S. Department of Military Medicine (Singh and Day 1989) on Navy Sea, Air and Land (SEAL) Trainees. After the SEALs completed a week of intense physical training—involving hand-to-hand combat, underwater demolition, sleep deprivation, and much more—the levels of trace elements (for example, zinc and copper) found in their blood had dropped by 20 to 40 percent. These trace elements specifically relate to problems such as insomnia, loss of bone density, and the weakening of connective tissues. (The study asserted that the psychological stresses endured by the SEALs contributed to further depletion—an important fact for competitive athletes.) Replacing the lost micronutrients through diet alone would be a major planning challenge, compounded by a lack of micronutrient guidance from the DRIs, which are still evolving. In light of this study and other evidence, athletes who train hard with their eyes on elite status should consider the potential value of performance-enhancing products.

Some athletes question the value of any food that didn't sprout from dirt or have a mother. In contrast, others think, "More is better," when it comes to bars, shakes, and other supplemental items. If you can get a bar with 30 grams of protein, why eat one that has only 23? In fact, why eat one, when you can eat two? If you can get a drink that's 12 percent carbohydrates, why drink one that's only 8 percent? This line of thought leads to the questions—and answers—explored in the upcoming chapters.

Questions about the correct, or ideal, use of sports foods arise for many reasons, and they are fueled by mixed messages from clinical studies as much as from product claims in ads and testimonials from other athletes. The questions can and will be answered, and the place to start is by looking at the thinking behind the different categories of products.

Endurance: The Goal That Launched an Industry

Canadian Brian Maxwell was a world-class marathoner by the mid-1970s and ranked third internationally in 1977. As the long-distance running coach at the University of California, Berkeley, he had a schedule and an environment that let him explore his personal best. By 1983, he had won

14 marathons and earned the distinction of Canadian national champion four times. Throughout this competitive period, Brian explored ways that nutrition would help him shave minutes from his time and stave off stomach distress. He explains,

> It had always been my experience that if I had a problem in my running, it was something to do with my stomach. It was always a concern of either running out of energy, or eating something too close to competition, or eating the wrong thing and upsetting my stomach. I would have to stop and go to the bathroom or throw up. I had made a choice for a couple of years in my career that, rather than risk stomach upset, I would rather be on the empty side.

Most marathons began in the early morning, so Brian would simply wake up, show up, and run. He relied on the carbohydrate-loading ritual he used before competitions to meet his energy needs without breakfast. In the six-day period before a race, he would endure three days of carbohydrate depletion followed by three days of high-carb intake, and that regimen worked well—most of the time. He wasn't at all prepared for how a lack of food would cripple him in a race that started at noon.

Carbohydrate Loading: The Old-Fashioned Solution

Depleting the glycogen in the muscles—"hitting the wall," or "bonking"—can be a problem for athletes who train or compete for more than 90 minutes at a stretch. Before products were available to help athletes reload muscle glycogen stores quickly, top competitors commonly used carbohydrate loading to boost their muscle glycogen stores before a marathon, triathlon, or similar event. Many still do a version of the regimen with or without the addition of performance-enhancing foods.

The classic way to carb load was a six-day program that began with a high-intensity training session—for a marathoner, it might be a 20-mile run—and three days of a low- or no-carbohydrate diet. During those three days, the athletes would continue to train and, as a result, bring muscle glycogen stores to an extremely low level. In many cases, this practice would literally make the athletes sick. The onset of hypoglycemia (low blood sugar) and ketosis (increased blood acids) meant nausea, dizziness, bad temper, and fatigue. For the next three days before competition, the athletes rested and ate carbohydrates. The result could easily be a doubling of muscle glycogen stores, plenty of energy to complete the event.

(continued)

A newer method of carbohydrate loading begins with the athletes exercising intensely for about 90 minutes on day one and eating a diet of 50 percent carbohydrates. On the next two days, they reduce the workout to 40-minute sessions and stick with the same level of carbs in the daily diet. On the following two days, they bump up carb intake to about 70 percent and reduce activity to 20-minute workouts. On the final day before the competition, the athletes rest and maintain the high-carb diet. The result matches that of the classic carbohydrate loading program.

After he led until mile 20 of the 26.2-mile race, Brian's energy slowed to a trickle. Finishing seventh, he returned to Berkeley with the idea that there had to be some food or drink that was perfect for endurance, something that could be consumed right before a race that wouldn't make a runner sick. He figured there had to be something better than 1972 Olympic gold medalist Frank Shorter's "secret formula"—Coca-Cola that had lost its fizz, a tasty blend of caffeine, sugar, and colored water.

Over the course of many months, Brian took his clipboard to running and cycling events and asked about 2,000 endurance athletes to fill out a nutrition survey. Questions included the following: What do you eat before you compete? How active are you? What foods work for you? Brian discovered that oatmeal and other grain products, as well as some fruits, seemed to work best before a race.

His research led him and a biochemist friend, Dr. William Vaughan, to attempt to create an energy bar. They started off with a set of guidelines about what they did not want in a bar, as well as a set of ingredients that they did want. Fats—especially saturated fats—led the "no" list, which also included lactose and caffeine. Fats slow digestion; lactose causes stomach distress in some adults; and caffeine, despite the kick it may provide, dehydrates the body. The two men did want to include grains, so they researched which grains were least likely to stimulate allergic reactions. Oats and rice topped the "yes" list. Next Brian and Bill found an independent manufacturer that made candy bars on contract. The management promised, "Give us your guidelines, and we'll formulate a bar for you." Brian recalls,

> When we showed them our guidelines, they said, "Here's the problem. You say you don't want any saturated fat, but you have to understand, that's how bar products are made. If you want to make a bar product, you start with a highly saturated fat, like palm kernel oil or lard. It has to be solid at room temperature and liquid at warmer temperatures. We start with oil, and then add sugar.

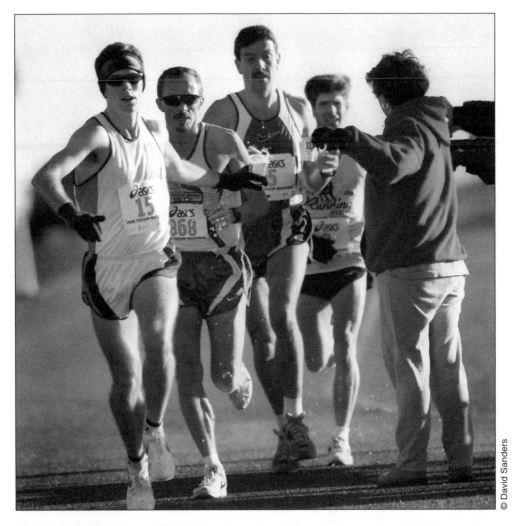

© David Sanders

Runners struggle to find foods that provide quick energy without causing stomach distress.

That forms the matrix that holds the bar together. After that, you can add whatever healthy stuff you want."

Brian left the plant determined to find a way to make a completely healthy bar that delivered sustained energy. As George Bernard Shaw once observed, "The reasonable man adapts himself to the world; the unreasonable man persists in trying to adapt the world to himself. Therefore, all progress depends on the unreasonable man."

Brian did not have instant success in trying to prove the bar manufacturers wrong. That night, he went into his kitchen and mixed a concoction of milk powder, ground-up breakfast cereal, apple juice, and crushed vitamin pills. It turned into a paste, which he left out on a pan. There it dried into glop. Brian cautiously tasted it and declared it a disaster.

He read a study about oat bran and learned that it was a soluble fiber and natural sort of gel. Suddenly oat bran was his Holy Grail, but the quest for it presented a bigger problem than he'd expected. In 1983, oat bran wasn't considered human food. He could only get it from a supplier that provided feed for horses. Armed with a 100-pound bag, he went back into the kitchen. He theorized that he might be able to use a combination of oat bran and rice flour together with water and fructose syrup to create a stable bar-shaped food. Fructose, the main type of sugar in fruit and the sweetener of choice for many diabetics, does not stimulate dramatic insulin release as other sugars do.

About this time, Jennifer Biddulph entered the picture. A runner as well as a nutrition and food science student at Berkeley, she helped Brian tinker with the formula and wrapped the results in plastic for their running and cycling friends. Based on the responses of people to whom they gave the bar, Brian and Jennifer kept coming closer to a workable formula. In the early days, many ate it and ran like they'd never run before—to the bathroom. By 1986, athletes were offering to pay for the bar of fructose, oat bran, maltodextrins, milk proteins, vitamins, minerals, and amino acids. Athletes dubbed it a "powerful bar." Brian and Jennifer called it PowerBar, the first of its kind.

Training Your Head to Use Sports Foods

Designed with the energy needs of endurance athletes in mind, the original PowerBar was eventually joined on the shelves by direct competitors as well as products addressing different aims—energy bursts, recovery, weight gain, weight loss, aid for damaged joints, and more. Sports foods offer some unique benefits in all these areas and even provide shortcuts to achieving athletic goals. Some athletes may be tempted to use the products as substitutes for training and real food instead of supplements to them. A marathoner, for example, may compensate for insufficient or incorrect training by sucking down carbohydrate gel every five miles. World-class runners know that periodic sessions of 18 miles or more can train the body to use fat as fuel after muscle glycogen stores have dwindled. If they do use gels, which digest easily and convert to glycogen in just a couple minutes, they do so late in the race. Many people running marathons today have a much less ambitious regimen; consequently their bodies need fuel they can absorb easily throughout the race. Some of these people get to the finish line, but it's a safe bet they don't lead the pack.

Some athletes try to use these products as a substitute for whole food because of their desire to eat the "right" amount of macronutrients and micronutrients. If an envelope of protein powder says that the product delivers 42 grams of protein, 25 grams of carbohydrates, 2 grams of fat, and 50 percent of all major vitamins and minerals, an athlete may wonder, "Why bother eating meat and vegetables?" That envelope takes the guesswork—the thinking, actually—out of food choices. Aside from a couple of folks on the fringes of good sense, even the people who developed these foods readily admit that no one should try to live on them. A steady diet of designer foods will result in deficiencies. In addition to being important entertainment for the taste buds, a balanced diet provides arrays of nutrients that allow the supplemental foods to kick athletes into high gear. Most importantly, hundreds of phytochemicals in fruits and vegetables have benefits that are not yet captured adequately in supplement form.

Nonetheless, the eating regimens structured to support the goals of some athletes are anything but balanced. Bodybuilders top the list of athletes who deliberately and routinely adopt imbalanced diets. Sports foods can play a key role in keeping these athletes healthy during cycles of their training when their eating habits would typically become aberrant.

For decades, bodybuilders adhered to stringent diets built on anecdotal evidence from other athletes and the nutritional knowledge of their trainers. In the mid-1980s, serious bodybuilders typically ate lean beef, chicken breasts, fish, egg whites—none of these ever fried, of course—citrus fruit, and possibly dry baked potatoes and pasta with no sauce. That was not just the usual diet; it was the entire diet for months at a time. Acceptable drinks included distilled water, coffee, tea, and an occasional cup of skim milk. Imagine the joy, and the unrestrained cash outlays, when low-fat, high-protein products that tasted good finally hit the health food stores.

Besides adding variety to the diet of weight-training athletes, these products had the ability to help avert health problems. Just as endurance athletes devoted to a classic carb loading program before competition would experience hypoglycemia and ketosis during the carb-depletion phase, bodybuilders commonly made themselves sick dieting for shows. Misguided by a superstition that carbohydrates of any kind added to body fat, some competitors tried to live on little more than boiled chicken breasts until the day of the show.

Fortunately, weight-training athletes can now rely on many products to boost the development of lean muscle mass while maintaining their strength and health. Unfortunately, in response to the enormous market demand, the choices are so numerous that athletes often select a product based solely on the endorsement of a top athlete in their sport, on the amount of protein in the product, or on a taste-test—none of which is a reliable way to assess the merits of a product. For example, bars that taste like candy often have more saturated fat than the others. A typical selection of bars aimed at athletes striving for lean mass might include MET-Rx's Big 100, SportPharma's Promax, American Body Building Products' Steel Bar, EAS's Myoplex Plus Deluxe, Labrada Bodybuilding Nutrition's Lean Body, and Worldwide Sport Nutrition's Pure Protein. They are all protein bars for weight-training athletes, and they all have approximately the same number of calories (300), but the amount of saturated fat ranges from .5 grams to 4.0 grams—eight times the amount of the low-fat item.

The bars higher in fat take longer to digest; they are generally not the food you want just prior to a workout. On the other hand, some relatively high-fat bars are also high-quality bars, so they may earn a place somewhere in your diet. You may also want to consider whether a product includes ingredients that could cause water retention. The subsequent chapters will help you sort out considerations like this about the full range of products for energy, recovery, strength, weight loss, and so on— products that now number in the hundreds (or the thousands, if you count different flavors). Before you leap into the world of performance-enhancing products, however, prepare your body to make the most of them: establish a balanced base diet.

The Basis for Supplements: An Athlete's Diet

Many dedicated, well-informed athletes push common sense right out of the locker room when it comes to nutrition. They develop superstitions about food, put too much faith in trainers or doctors who may have their own superstitions, or model their diets after the athletes at the top of their sport.

Steps to Enhancing Performance Through Nutrition

Your dietary goal as an athlete is to develop energy for useful purposes rather than pointless storage mechanisms. You want your eating to support a fine-tuned metabolism.

- Eat an athlete's diet—a balance of macronutrients.
- Adjust the amount of carbohydrates, protein, and fat according to sport, training cycle, and personal responses.
- Add sports foods to get an edge in training and competition.
- Add micronutrients to sharpen the edge.

- Monitor shifts in performance; move to new or different sports foods and supplements as needed.
- Don't get superstitious—bodies do change, products can improve, and new studies can point the way to better answers.

Both the science and the common sense of nutrition flow from a paradox: We are all different, but we are all the same. As humans, we share physiological traits that relate to our dietary needs: Some foods seem to be very good for the human body, whereas the body simply tolerates other foods. For example, the body can process refined sugar, but it cannot be described as "very good" for any of us. MET-Rx founder Scott Connelly, MD, who now specializes in the nutritional needs of athletes, came out of a critical care environment. His research in human metabolism helped develop supplements and dietary programs for patients wasting away from illness. Early in his research, he looked at human evolution for clues about what people should eat, and as a corollary, what foods people should avoid. As Dr. Connelly concluded,

> There is no magical disconnect between evolution and metabolism. Our brain size and complexity reflect billions of years of evolution, but the liver is the same liver as 10,000 years ago when agriculture came into being. It's impossible to suggest that any significant genetic change has occurred at the level of metabolism to account and deal with the perversion of the natural food supply that has occurred, first and foremost with agriculture. On top of that, 200 years ago industrialization brought processing into the picture. All of this has added up to task the system beyond its limits for metabolic transformation.

The first guideline to come out of research such as Dr. Connelly's is to avoid processed foods whenever possible. It's normal to have cake at weddings or a few cookies at Christmas. It is damaging to your athletic performance to eat these white flour/white sugar treats on a regular basis.

You may think it's ironic that a book devoted to foods and drinks developed in laboratories would condemn processed foods. "Processed foods" in this context means foods that were stripped of much of their original nutritional value. "Enriched processed foods" are processed foods with vitamins and minerals added to them in the manufacturing plant, such as many breads and cereals. I don't recommend them, either. "Enriched foods," on the other hand, are foods that haven't undergone much processing; the vendor added vitamins or minerals to help consumers meet daily needs. A common example is calcium-fortified orange juice. When I refer to "engineered foods," I mean those designed specifically to enhance your performance. If you want the full benefits of foods and supplements designed specifically to help you be a better athlete, you must start with a clean base diet that helps regulate key body functions such as insulin release and fat metabolism. Anything made with bleached flour and sugar has no place in that diet.

Dr. Barry Sears, who developed the "Zone diet" and has helped Olympians such as Dara Torres achieve gold-medal performance levels, says the importance of a good base diet centers on hormonal control:

> The real power of nutrition is its ability to alter hormones, and that becomes the key to reaching your full performance potential as an athlete. From the standpoint of an athlete, there are certain hormones that we know to be beneficial in terms of building muscle mass. There are certain hormones that are beneficial in terms of increasing oxygen transfer. Those are the hormones you want to be orchestrating, using your food as if it were a drug.

Barry's approach in the Zone diet is therefore focused on two hormones—insulin and eicosanoids that he sees as most related to oxygen transfer, blood sugar levels, inflammation, muscle mass, and the accessibility of stored body fat as an energy source. He cautions athletes that insulin is controlled by the ratio of protein to carbohydrates at every meal and eicosanoids are controlled by the ratio of omega-3 to omega-6 fats (Sears 1995).

Whether you go for the Zone diet or another program, forget the Food Pyramid. Think of a Food Circle (figure 1.1) in which the largest area is devoted to water. As an athlete, you want to do whatever it takes to avoid dehydration. Even a mild dehydration can slow your metabolism as much as 3 percent and cause some degree of fatigue.

The fats you eat should not exceed 30 percent of your diet. Other than that, how you determine the percentages of the macronutrients—fats, protein, and carbohydrates—should not be a prescription from someone who doesn't even know your body. You, and possibly your coach or trainer, are the most tuned in to your energy, weight, strength, and body composition goals.

Here are some guidelines for building your unique daily diet. Start with water and water-rich, unprocessed foods—fruits and vegetables. Add slightly less than a gram of protein for every pound of bodyweight, or roughly two grams for every kilogram. This includes vegetable sources of protein, such as nuts and legumes (soybeans, lentils, kidney beans, etc.). Put in some fiber-rich grains that make great side dishes, breakfast items, and soup ingredients—oats, kasha, quinoa, millet, amaranth, and

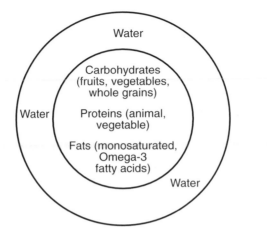

Figure 1.1   Food Circle.

barley. To keep your meals interesting and your cholesterol count in line, add small amounts of good fat, or monounsaturated fats, such as olive oil, and be sure to include sources of omega-3 fat, such as cold-water fish and flax seed.

To some people, these guidelines might appear ridiculously stringent. If you're in that camp, consider the ways modern society has made it easier, not harder, to eat well.

• Frozen fruits and vegetables aren't exactly processed. Actually, because they are subjected to flash freezing immediately after harvest, they can be good substitutes for fresh produce. In fact, sometimes frozen produce is better than fresh, which may sit on a truck for a few days before it even gets to your grocery store. Just read the labels and avoid the packages that indicate added sugar or some distortion of the natural food.

• Canned sardines, tuna, and salmon can definitely have a place in an athlete's diet. Just be sure that you get the varieties packed in water, not oil.

• There is such a thing as good bread that serves as a convenient source of whole-grain benefits, but it's usually not white bread. The refining process that makes white wheat flour removes the outer coating (the bran) and the wheat germ, which is the seed of the new plant. Since 90 percent of the fiber comes from the bran and germ, even bread fortified with vitamins and minerals can be low in fiber, which your body absolutely needs for peak efficiency. Read the label; when the list of ingredients begins with enriched flour and moves on to cottonseed oil and sugar, find another loaf.

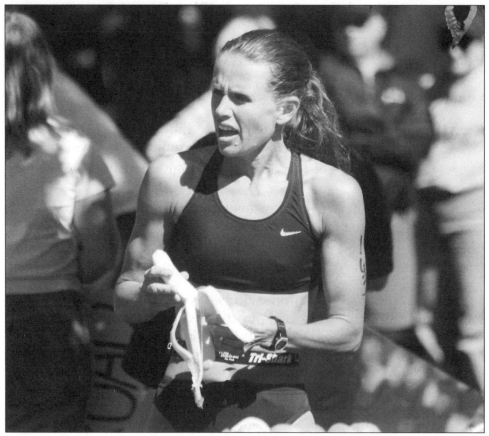

© iphotonews.com/Brooks

Athletes need fresh fruits and vegetables to reach peak performance.

And what about having a couple beers during the football game or meeting your gym buddies at Starbucks for a latté?

• You can enjoy alcohol, but it can affect your metabolism, your sleep, your hydration, and your need for certain vitamins and minerals. The question, Should I drink? is best answered by another question: How good do you want to be at your sport?

• If you must, go ahead and have your coffee, but put limits on the caffeine intake so you don't risk dehydration or diarrhea or throw off your energy balance. An acceptable level of caffeine is about 3 milligrams per kilogram of bodyweight, or 1.5 milligrams per pound. A cup of coffee contains about 120 milligrams of caffeine, so a normal adult should be able to handle that without getting dizzy or jittery. In fact, according to the formula, a 150-pound adult should be able to have a couple of cups of coffee (or the equivalent in another beverage or sports gel) without any problem. More than that amount usually makes no sense in terms of athletic performance or health.

A Tool for Control: The Food Log

If you want to get serious about developing the best diet for yourself and using performance-enhancing foods to their greatest advantage, be consistent about your eating and keep a log. In your log, make notes about your athletic performance:

- How does the diet work on routine training days? During high-intensity or extra-long sessions? On competition days?
- How do you feel the day after a high-intensity or extra-long session?
- Keep track of your energy level throughout the day. Do you ever have big fluctuations in energy?
- Pay attention to the quality of your sleep. Do you feel rested after six hours one day, but groggy after eight hours another?

These important observations will help you see where performance-enhancing products could make a difference, in terms of both your carbohydrate-protein-fat balance and your intake of vitamins and minerals. They can also tell you something about your sources of nutrition—some foods might cause slight stomach distress or make you feel sluggish.

What are the macronutrient percentages you are likely to settle on? Depending on your body, your sport, and your genes, they could vary considerably. One split that grew in popularity because of the Zone diet is a 40-30-30 diet (carbohydrates-protein-fat). The Zone diet itself, however, is far more than simple ratios. It involves making food choices with hormonal control in mind; your carb source would never be chocolate cake. Some athletes don't like a 40-30-30 diet because it doesn't seem to provide them with enough quick energy from carbohydrates. They prefer the USDA-suggested amounts, which start at 55 to 65 percent carbohydrates, include about 20 to 25 percent protein, and keep fat to 20 percent or less. Others don't feel either of these macronutrient splits serves their aim of building lean muscle mass or staying energetic in their sport, so they opt for a diet consistent with Scott Connelly's evolution-based thinking: a high-protein, relatively high-fiber program that is very low in fat. This is a common choice for bodybuilders. To some extent, the split may depend on what kind of athlete you are, what training cycle you're in, and even what gives you a psychological boost.

To move closer to a diet that supports your training and event requirements for energy and strength, use a daily tracking form like the one on page 14 combined with a log containing notes about how you feel and perform. Be sure to include in the log any supplements, energy products,

Nutrition Tracking Form

Day of the week: _____   Date:_____

Qty. meas.	Food item	Protein (gm)	Carbs (gm)	Fat (gm)	Total calories
	Subtotals				
	Caloric multiplier	X 4	X 4	X 9	
	Calculated calories				
	Percent total calories	%	%	%	
	Approximate goals	%	%	%	

Courtesy of Ric Giardina, founder of *Spirit Employed.*

and other performance-enhancing foods you use. A potential benefit is that you may be able to avoid crippling problems during competition. For example, if you've been relying on a carbohydrate drink for six months, but one day during your workout you get cramps, jot that down. You've clearly done something different with your diet or training regimen (for example, a change in altitude) to cause that negative result. If you can't identify the source of the problem by looking at your daily tracking form, maybe you'll figure it out the next time it happens. At that point, you'll be able to compare your eating and drinking patterns from two different blocks of time, which might make the cause of the problem obvious.

Performance-enhancing foods are helping athletes excel beyond their heroes in many activities and events. Long-standing records are now falling, in part because more athletes know how to use engineered foods to give them an edge. But until technology can capture all of the goodness and value of real foods, athletes who want to reach their full potential must look at sports foods as merely supplemental to what nature provides.

CHAPTER 2

Eating for Energy

For years, athletes thought that candy was the ideal quick-energy source and steak was a good pre-competition meal. Those misperceptions are changing, in part because foods designed to deliver energy have proven their worth. This chapter explores why and how eating habits are changing and investigates the link between sport-specific energy needs and different products, ranging from those that deliver sustained energy to those that give a short-lived kick.

A little bit of background about how your body uses food to generate energy will prepare you to make smart choices about energy products. Ingredients and product claims will make more sense to you. Best of all, the information will help you avoid wasting money on foods, drinks, and supplements designed for some other athlete in some other sport.

Energy Basics:
Where Does Energy Come From?

The energy equation is

$$\text{food} + \text{oxygen} = \text{carbon dioxide } (CO_2), \text{ water } (H_2O),$$
$$\text{and adenosine triphosphate (ATP)}.$$

That means you have to eat and you have to breathe to make energy. ATP is the body's direct energy supply, a chemical substance required for all muscular activity. Energy can either be used by the body for various functions or be liberated as heat. If there's anything left, the body tries to store it in one of two "compartments"—fat or muscle. Athletes must figure out how to get the greatest benefits from stored energy (that is, how to store it in the form of functional or structural tissue components).

Your body uses energy continuously, whether you are training or sleeping. There is no "off" switch that tells body processes to shut down and wait for the next supply of food. Among other requirements, your body continuously needs blood glucose (blood sugar) to run the brain, the heart, and the kidneys. If you don't eat in a way that provides the necessary raw materials to your biochemical factories, they get them from other places in the body. The tissue that's affected most is muscle. Your muscle already has huge responsibilities for keeping the body healthy—it's the only source of stored nitrogen, which is vital for basic functions like cell division—so asking it to make up for deficits in eating means loss of athletic ability. A basic concept in eating for energy, therefore, is that *the food you eat must serve your entire body's need for fuel, down to the cellular level.* It's more than a matter of routinely slamming down a drink laced with ephedrine and caffeine and then charging into the gym.

Carbohydrates, proteins, and fats all play a role in energy production. Carbohydrates, as the name implies, are made up of carbon and water (and water is hydrogen and oxygen, or H_2O). Fat is also composed of carbon, oxygen, and hydrogen, but it has a different molecular structure. Proteins, which consist of amino acids, have these three elements plus nitrogen and, in many cases, sulfur. (Arginine and alanine are examples of amino acids that do not contain sulfur.) The latter elements set it apart from the other nutrients in the role it plays in body functions.

Carbohydrates are a ready source of fuel for both the body and the brain. The simplest form of carbohydrates is the *simple sugars*—glucose, fructose, and galactose. These sugars bind together in various combinations to form different kinds of complex carbohydrates. Your body breaks down the complex carbohydrates into glucose—it's the main sugar in your blood and serves as your basic body fuel.

What Is "Hitting the Wall"?

Glycogen is glucose that's stored in your muscles and liver. Each gram of glycogen contains four calories of energy. The average person stores between 1,500 and 2,000 calories, which is enough fuel for a 20-mile run for most athletes. Consider how common it is for athletes to "hit the wall"—in technical terms, deplete their muscle glycogen stores—at about the 20-mile mark. This is about the time when even elite athletes turn to a food product that quickly raises their blood sugar to keep them going. That fuel intake is important for more than the muscle movement. The brain relies on blood glucose as its main fuel and has essentially no stored supply.

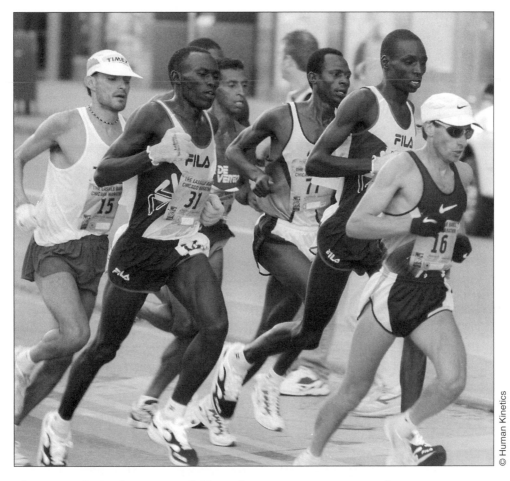

© Human Kinetics

Choose carbohydrates carefully to keep your energy steady.

Although all carbohydrates break down into glucose, which carbohydrates you choose makes an enormous difference in how energetic you feel for a workout or competition. This is because *different carbohydrates, whether they're simple or complex, do not give your body the same results in terms of energy.* This important concept ties in with the recommendations made later, in the chapter on energy products.

Without carbohydrates in the system, the body turns to protein and fat as sources of energy. The scenario of your body having to use protein for fuel is not ideal, because having your protein diverted from its main jobs can cause you to lose muscle mass and strength. First and foremost, dietary protein replenishes proteins in the body that have essential life-supporting functions. You need proteins for muscle growth and repair, for the formation of new tissues, and for fighting diseases, because antibodies and other elements supported by the immune system are proteins.

The Glycemic Index: A Key to Understanding Energy Foods

The glycemic index (GI) rates foods according to how fast they raise your blood sugar level. It was created to help people with diabetes select foods that didn't result in an insulin spike, but it's extremely useful for athletes as well.

Anytime you eat carbohydrates when your body is at rest, your blood glucose rises. In turn, insulin production and secretion escalate. Your pancreas releases insulin, a hormone, into the bloodstream after you eat. It helps cells absorb the sugars (carbs), fatty acids, and amino acids (elements of protein) so that your body can synthesize protein, increase the energy reserve in your muscles, and store fat.

In doing its job, insulin acts to lower blood glucose concentration. For training or competing, you want to maintain a steady blood glucose level or your performance will suffer. You don't want a high insulin level to drive down your blood sugar when you need to feel energetic.

Foods that have a low glycemic index don't cause a dramatic release of insulin. Conversely, foods with a high GI will send insulin rushing into your bloodstream. The exception is during exercise, because the insulin response to eating carbohydrates is suppressed when you're active. Foods all along the GI spectrum have a role in your diet and in your sports foods.

- Low GI foods include beans, barley, cherries, and grapefruit.
- Moderate GI foods include some sustained-energy bars. It also includes such foods as pita bread, apricots, pineapples, and corn. Energy bars with a somewhat higher fat content may fall into this category because the fat slows the absorption of sugar in your system.
- High GI foods include quick-energy foods such as white potatoes, pasta, many popular cereals, crackers, most cookies, cakes, and similar foods with processed sugar. There is a definite time and place for high GI foods and products. By design, energy gels tend to be on the high side, although even gels can have very different GI ratings. Chapter 10 contains a sidebar about sweeteners that helps clarify these differences.

All enzymes and a number of hormones are also proteins, so they are also critical for many body processes. It's the sequence of the amino acids in a protein that determines what particular job it will have in body processes.

Fats play an important role in body functions as well. You need fats to metabolize the fat-soluble vitamins A, D, E, and K, so dietary fat has value. Dietary fat doesn't have to come in the form of added fat, though. The plants and animals that supply your body with carbohydrates and proteins contain fat naturally. Since fat provides nine calories per gram versus the four calories per gram you get from carbohydrates and protein, it would appear to be a great energy source. But dietary fat slows your digestion, so foods formulated to deliver quick energy invariably have a very low or zero fat content. Unlike consumed fat, fat stored in the body is a great source of energy for long-distance runners, cyclists, and other endurance athletes; your body converts *any* food to stored fat if it has an energy surplus. Through diligent efforts, you can determine how much of each food source to consume so that your body is trained to keep stored fat to an acceptable level and draw on it when the need arises.

Energy Systems

Three different energy systems supply your muscles with the energy you get from food. Which one kicks in depends on the nature and duration of the activity you're doing. Two of the systems are anaerobic, which means they produce ATP without oxygen being present, and one is aerobic, which means it requires oxygen. When you are resting or doing any activity in which your body's need for oxygen is easily met, the aerobic energy system is at work. When you are doing an activity like heavy weightlifting or biking up a steep hill, and your body can't meet the demand for oxygen to produce ATP, it relies on the anaerobic energy systems. You can get great bursts of energy from your anaerobic systems, but that energy won't last long. For any activity that requires sustained energy, you need your aerobic system.

Figure 2.1 shows how your body goes to the anaerobic systems when you have an acute need for energy. When your need is at a peak, your body breaks down creatine phosphate, an amino acid, to resupply ATP to the muscles. The phosphocreatine system delivers a great boost, but the ATP supplied from it is depleted after 8 to 10 seconds of all-out activity. The lactic acid system, which is also anaerobic, sustains you through slightly longer periods of intense need—like a round in a boxing match or a set of squats. For the long haul, you must be working in the aerobic zone most of the time.

In a number of sports, you will use all three systems at different times during your training or competition. The energy system that dominates depends on your activity—how intense it is and how long it lasts.

Some evidence suggests that creatine supplements can boost the body's reserves of usable creatine, enhancing recovery between

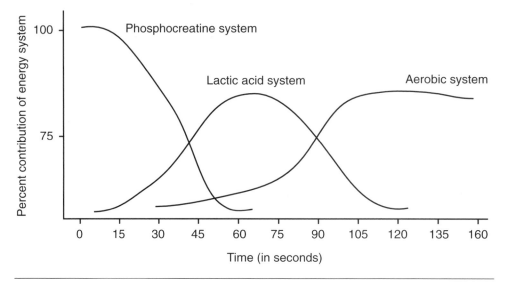

Figure 2.1 The three systems that supply your muscles with energy.

short periods of high intensity exercise. As a corollary, it can potentially aid the development of muscle mass, which is addressed in chapter 4. (See the sidebar on creatine loading.)

Creatine Loading: Feeding the Body's Quick-Energy System

The theory behind creatine loading, a one-week program of high dosages of creatine, is that you want to get as much creatine into your body as it can hold to create energy/recovery advantages. Loading may not be the only way to accomplish this saturation (Stout et al. 2000); FSI Nutrition maintains that its patented effervescent creatine formula seems to achieve saturation without loading. If you have a noneffervescent creatine monohydrate product you like using, how-ever, and you want to gauge the effect of loading on your performance, here are some guidelines.

Athletes who require bursts of intense energy and power, such as power lifters and football players, are good candidates for loading. Endurance athletes are not, because the loading causes muscle tissue to retain excess fluid. If you're a marathon runner or alpine climber, this result could compromise your performance. It's better for endurance athletes who use creatine to stick with the normal recommended dosage of .03 to .06 grams per kilogram of bodyweight (approximately .015 to .03 grams per pound), or about two to five grams per day for most athletes. (The variance reflects the fact that clinical tests involving creatine are ongoing; some suggest staying at the lower end of the range for a maintenance dose, whereas others suggest that a slightly higher dosage is better.)

Loading is designed to increase muscle creatine content by roughly 20 percent. It is also associated with the development of fat-free mass, an application discussed in chapter 4.

Products that feature creatine monohydrate, which helps the body produce the form it needs for energy, come in powders, serums, gels, drinks, capsules, and tablets. Not all of them are well suited for creatine loading. As mentioned previously, the effervescent creatine patented by FSI is not a loading product; according to the company, it is designed to achieve saturation through steady use. Creatine serum is also not suited for creatine loading. Regardless of the form in which you take it, expect to pay about $10 per day for creatine products during a loading program.

Precisely how much you take during the loading period depends on your weight, with the usual load being four times the normal daily amount, or about 20 grams per day. Paul Greenhaff, PhD, who conducts creatine research at the University of Nottingham in England, recommends taking four doses of five grams each, accompanied each time by 100 grams of high-GI carbs such as baked potatoes or pasta. The carbs seem to help transport the creatine to the muscles and to boost significantly the amount they retain.

Pay attention to the amount of creatine in one serving of the product you choose so that you don't waste it. Most powders, for example, deliver more than five grams. EAS's PhosphoGain has eight grams in a serving and several others have six grams. If you take more than you need, your urine will contain the excess.

Follow these guidelines when you use creatine:

- Take the creatine about an hour before your training session so that it's in your bloodstream during the workout. Some products designed for quick energy and recovery also contain creatine, which may be fine—whether or not it makes sense depends on the other ingredients in the formula. Remember that high-GI carbs seem to promote creatine transport.

- When the week-long loading period is over, stop the loading and move to a maintenance dosage. Once you achieve muscle saturation, a maintenance dosage should be all you need to maintain saturated tissue levels of creatine. Anything more is a waste of your money.

(continued)

- Creatine loading can dehydrate you. Drink a lot of extra water during the program: about two ounces for each kilogram of bodyweight (or a little less than one ounce per pound).
- A 1996 study determined that caffeine cancels creatine's performance benefit. Don't waste the creatine by washing it down with a cup of coffee, a Red Bull, Mountain Dew, Ripped Force, or any other caffeinated drink (Vandenberghe et al.).
- Some people experience bloating, gas, cramping, diarrhea, or a combination of all these symptoms when they load. Try increasing your fluid intake to alleviate the symptoms, and if that doesn't help, reduce your dosage.
- Experiment with loading during a hard training cycle. Don't inaugurate the practice just before a competition.

The second anaerobic system, which supplies rapid energy for up to about three minutes, is called the lactic acid system. As an athlete, you have undoubtedly experienced the effects of accumulated lactic acid—aching, fatigue, and possibly muscle failure. Many athletes actually enjoy the pain that reflects a heavy training day. Pleasant or unpleasant, these outcomes are the result of placing energy requirements on the lactic acid system, which produces ATP through the incomplete breakdown of carbohydrates. Needless to say, the operation of this system depends on carbohydrates. Keep this in mind as the various energy products are examined later in this chapter.

Many weight-training athletes in particular, seem to think that protein bars, powders, and drinks should be their fuel source going into the gym. In reality, they will be calling upon their lactic acid energy system throughout the workout and would be better served by a preworkout carbohydrate boost.

The mother lode of energy is the aerobic system, which has the capacity to produce ATP for long periods of time. This system can only function when you are training or competing at a submaximal level, however; that is, your body has to be getting enough oxygen to continue the activity. As soon as you move to a more intense level at which your oxygen needs cannot be met, the anaerobic systems kick in. At that point, you either have to move back into the aerobic zone or face an energy shutdown. The aerobic system uses all sources of energy—carbohydrates, proteins, and, eventually, stored fat.

Common Ground:
Energy Food Considerations for All Athletes

You should eat or drink a carbohydrate snack before your workouts to ensure that you have two sources of energy: blood glucose (blood sugar) and muscle glycogen (sugar stored in the muscle). The question is, how long before? "One formula suggests that you should ingest 1 gm per kg of your bodyweight an hour before exercise," (Dorfman 2000). The complete answer also depends on the composition of the product and on whether you ingest it in a liquid, solid, or gel form. During exercise, blood goes to your muscles. You don't have a lot of blood going to your intestines, so it's difficult to digest food. If your exercise is an intense cardiorespiratory workout or event, the digestion problem becomes acute. When your heart rate escalates to 70 or 75 percent of maximum and stays there, you are generating a lot of body heat in addition to using your muscles. Your body's primary function at that point is to maintain its core temperature, so your system very efficiently shunts blood to the surface of your body to dissipate heat. Your blood has vacated your gut so that you simply can't digest anything. The best you can hope for is a food that you can passively "absorb."

This biological process drives the design of energy foods and drinks for consumption before and during workouts. Many of these products have very little or no fat or protein, so that they are readily digestible. A good rule of thumb regarding energy bars is that the lower the amount of saturated fat they contain, the closer to workout time they can be comfortably consumed. A 230-calorie bar with two or three grams of unsaturated fat could be eaten less than 45 minutes before a workout. If you are extremely nervous about an event or workout, however, or if it's so intense that you will be stressing your strength or endurance to the maximum, these guidelines are not valid—your body will probably not be able to process food in a normal way. The type of workout you're doing, your metabolism, and the product's ingredients can all affect how you perform with the product.

Table 2.1 sheds light on the differences between some of these products. Note that it applies to routine workouts and not to the energy requirements associated with extraordinary situations, which are covered in later chapters.

Looking at the relatively high fat content in some of the bars—which is not necessarily bad, depending on your athletic goals—the question in your mind may be, how do these compare to my favorite Halloween candy? Whether you look at the bars in terms of ingredients or macronutrient profile can make a difference. You may see a non-sports-food bar

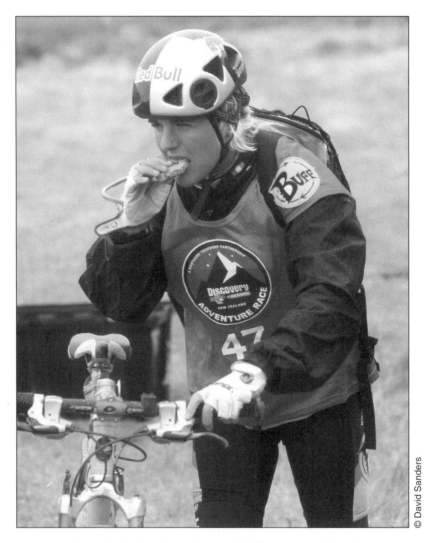

© David Sanders

Bars are convenient fuel, but be sure to drink water with them.

that approximates a 40-30-30 profile, but the fat may be primarily saturated, and the first or second ingredient in the list won't be soy protein
isolate, as it would in a PR Ironman or Zone Perfect bar. Another difference, although one of dubious significance in terms of your immediate
energy needs, is the addition of vitamins and minerals to the energy bar.

Where the bars really start to sound alike is in the description of the
chocolate coating. Here are the ingredients in the coating of one of the
energy bars covered in the chart: sugar, palm kernel oil, cocoa processed
with alkali, cocoa, whey powder, skim milk powder, soy lecithin, salt,
and vanilla extract. Compare that list to the ingredients in the coating of
a Snickers bar produced by Mars, Inc.: sugar, cocoa butter, chocolate,
lactose, skim milk, milk fat, soy lecithin, and artificial flavor.

Table 2.1 Energy Bar Chart: A Comparison of Nutrient Profiles and Best Uses

Product (company)	Calories (approx.)	Macronutrient profile (approx.) carb-protein-fat	Best use(s)	Comments
151 Bar— Fruit Burst Energy (Applied Nutrition/Omni Nutraceuticals)	230	80-5-15	Preworkout 30–45 min.; short duration	Uncoated; contains herbs
151 Bar— Peanut Butter Chocolate Protein Energy (Applied Nutrition/Omni Nutraceuticals)	290	50-15-35	Preworkout 1$\frac{1}{2}$–2 hr.; endurance	None
Balance (Balance Bar)	200	40-30-30	Preworkout 1$\frac{1}{2}$ hr.; endurance	None
Balance Gold (Balance Bar)	210	40-30-30	Preworkout 1$\frac{1}{2}$–2 hr.; endurance	More saturated fat than other Balance Bars
Balance Outdoor (Balance Bar)	200	40-30-30	Preworkout 1$\frac{1}{2}$–2 hr.; endurance	Uncoated
BodyBar (Score Athletic Products)	220	90-10-0	Preworkout 30–45 min.; short duration	None
Boulder Bar (Boulder Foods)	240	70-15-15	Preworkout 1–1$\frac{1}{2}$ hr.; endurance	Uncoated; vegan approved
Carbo-Crunch (Shaklee)	180	60-20-20	preworkout 1–1$\frac{1}{2}$ hr.; endurance	None
Clif (Clif Bar)	240	70-20-10	Preworkout 30–45 min.; endurance	Uncoated
E2R (TSI Supplements)	200	40-30-30	Preworkout 1$\frac{1}{2}$ hr.; endurance	None

(continued)

Table 2.1 *(continued)*

Product (company)	Calories (approx.)	Macronutrient profile (approx.) carb-protein-fat	Best use(s)	Comments
Edgebar (Nutritional N-ER-G Products)	220	75-15-10	Preworkout 45 min.–1 hr.; short duration	None
Energize (Nutripower)	144	90-10-0	Preworkout 30–45 min.; short duration	None
Energy Bar (York Barbell)	250	60-10-30	Preworkout 1½–2 hr.;	High in saturated fat
Energy Stick (SportsTech International)	120	70-15-15	Preworkout 1–1½ hr.; short duration	None
Energy to Go (Sun-Rype)	135	98-1-1	Preworkout 30–45 min.; short duration	Fruit in a wrapper
Extran Muesli (Royal Numico)	92	85-5-10	Preworkout 30–45 min.; short duration	Uncoated
Extreme Balance (Neways)	200	40-30-30	Preworkout 1–1½ hr.; endurance	None
Forza! (Universal)	230	75-20-5	Preworkout 30–45 min.; short duration	None
GatorBar (Gatorade)	220	90-5-5	Preworkout 30–45 min.; short duration	None
Maxim Fruit (Maxim)	180	90-5-5	Preworkout 30–45 min.; short duration	None
MealPack (Bear Valley)	400	55-15-30	Preworkout 1½–2 hr.; endurance	Eat half at a time, unless you are powering through 5,000 or more calories a day: uncoated

Product (company)	Calories (approx.)	Macronutrient profile (approx.) carb-protein-fat	Best use(s)	Comments
Odwalla Bar Super Protein (Odwalla)	260	70-20-10	Preworkout 1–1½ hr.; endurance	Uncoated
Odwalla Bar (Odwalla)	220	85-5-10	Preworkout 30–45 min.; short duration	Uncoated
Okanagan Sports Bar (Okanagan)	220	98-1-1	Preworkout 30–45 min.; short duration	Fruit in a wrapper
Parillo Energy Bar (Parillo)	230	60-25-15	Preworkout 1–1½ hr.; endurance	None
Peak Bar Fruit (Peak Bar)	285	80-5-15	Preworkout 45 min.–1 hr.; endurance	None
Performance Energy Bar (Performance)	220	75-20-5	Preworkout 30–45 min.; short duration	None
PowerBar Performance (PowerBar)	230	75-15-10	Preworkout 30–45 min.; short duration	Uncoated
PR Ironman (PR Nutrition)	230	40-30-30	Preworkout 1½–2 hr.; endurance	None
ProSports (MLO Products)	240	70-25-5	Preworkout 30–45 min.; short duration	None
PurePower (PurePower Sports Nutrition)	240	70-20-10	Preworkout 30–45 min.; short duration	None
SIS GO (Science in Sport)	220	80-15-5	Preworkout 30–45 min.; short duration	None
Source of Life Energy Bar (Nature's Plus)	180	45-25-30	Preworkout 1½–2 hr.; endurance	Contains herbs

(continued)

Table 2.1 *(continued)*

Product (company)	Calories (approx.)	Macronutrient profile (approx.) carb-protein-fat	Best use(s)	Comments
Tekno	280	85-10-5	Preworkout 30–45 min.; short duration	None
ThunderBar (Sports Pep)	220	80-15-5	Preworkout 30–45 min.; short duration	None
Tiger Sport (Weider Nutrition)	230	70-15-15	Preworkout 45 min.–1 hr.; short duration	None
Torque Bar	210	80-15-5	Preworkout 30–45 min.; short duration	None
Verve (Whole Foods)	210	80-15-5	Preworkout 30–45 min.; endurance	Uncoated
X-Trnr (Stim O Stam)	220	70-20-5	Preworkout 30–45 min.; short duration	None
Zone Perfect (Eicotech)	200	40-30-30	Preworkout $1^{1}/_{2}$–2hr.; endurance	None

There is good news in this. The manufacturer of the candy-bar clone is at least honest enough to list the ingredients.

As a complement or an alternative to energy bars, you might also consider a carbohydrate drink. These products feature slightly different carbohydrate sources, such as high fructose corn syrup, which is a very high-GI sugar, and glucose polymers, the term sometimes used for maltodextrins. Often used by endurance athletes before and during training and competition, these drinks are covered in chapter 5, "Adding Endurance." That chapter includes a table that offers the carbohydrate profiles of various products as well as recommendations for using them.

Another set of products focuses exclusively on delivering quick energy; the makers of these products aren't so concerned about the nutrient profile as they are about ingredients that cause an energy spike. On the labels, you'll see words like guarana seed, ma huang, and white willow bark. A close look at products containing such herbal stimulants—premixed drinks, capsules, and powders called thermogenic aids—is contained in chapter 6, "Gaining or Cutting Weight." Even though they are often used as quick-energy products, they were originally designed as diet aids, or fat-burning agents, and they continue to be associated primarily with that function.

Carbohydrate gels are also formulated for a nearly instant energy boost, as are products combining a small (1.5- to 2.5-gram) preworkout dose of creatine monohydrate with simple carbohydrates. Both of these products are relatively recent phenomena. They are generally for different audiences. Weight-training athletes might turn to creatine products for energy needs. (Refer to the sidebar earlier in this chapter for details about their use and potential value to energy and recovery. Other benefits of creatine are explored in chapter 4, "Supplementing for Strength.") In contrast, carbohydrate gels principally serve the needs of endurance athletes, by restoring glycogen levels during training or competition that exceeds an hour. It is interesting to note, however, that Olympic gold medal swimmer Dara Torres used GU—the first gel—in a loading program immediately prior to competition. She took one packet an hour and a half before a race, one packet 45 minutes before, and another 10 to 15 minutes before. Depending on the formula, gels can also help with muscle recovery after long exercise sessions.

Figure 2.2 tells you what ingredients to look for in different types of energy products and gives you the basics of matching types of these products to your performance needs.

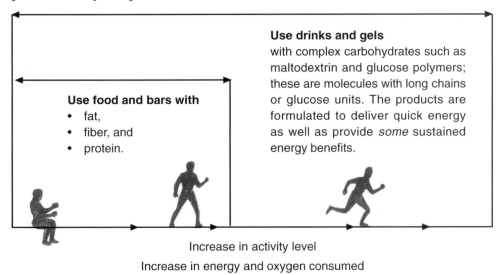

Use food and bars with
- fat,
- fiber, and
- protein.

Use drinks and gels
with complex carbohydrates such as maltodextrin and glucose polymers; these are molecules with long chains or glucose units. The products are formulated to deliver quick energy as well as provide *some* sustained energy benefits.

Increase in activity level
Increase in energy and oxygen consumed

Figure 2.2 Energy food during activities.
Courtesy of Sports Street Marketing.

The mind that created the first gel was not far, literally or physically, from the team that created the first energy bar. Actually, he was part of that genesis, too. When Brian Maxwell initially searched for a combination of ingredients that would deliver energy quickly, yet provide some sustained energy, his investigative partner was Dr. William Vaughan. With a PhD in biophysics and medical physics from the University of California at Berkeley, Bill brought extraordinary credentials to the effort that resulted in PowerBar. About five years after Brian and his colleague Jennifer Biddulph founded the company that introduced PowerBars to the sports world, Bill created another groundbreaking product: GU.

The impetus to formulate GU came when Bill saw his daughter, Laura, struggle to maintain her stamina while competing in a 100-mile race. Energy bars and drinks upset her stomach, but there were no alternatives. Bill headed to his lab. After several years of work with elite and recreational athletes, he formulated GU, a product intended to meet the following parameters:

- Never spoil
- Never freeze
- Digest quickly
- Boost energy quickly, but without leading to a sharp letdown
- Aid recovery by delaying buildup of lactic acid

By 1997, after a few competing products were developed to offer the same benefits, the energy gel market had grown to $10 million. An enormous surge in popularity occurred in the mid-1990s. Gels suddenly found a place in every endurance activity, from the Boston Marathon to Everest expeditions.

The gels are similar in many ways; this does not mean they are identical. Most gels share similar ingredients and other characteristics:

• Consistency. If you really care that your gel has the gooeyness of fudge sauce rather than the viscosity of icing that comes in a can, then squish the package before you buy it.

• Maltodextrin as a foundation ingredient. Maltodextrin is a complex carbohydrate that is easily absorbed from the gut; the glucose polymers of this substance deliver sustained energy.

• Fructose, or fruit sugar, as a main ingredient. Fructose is absorbed quickly, but your body utilizes it more slowly than glucose. (This is why many fruits fall into the medium-GI category as opposed to the high-GI category.)

• Branched chain amino acids (BCAAs). Many sports foods contain the BCAAs (leucine, isoleucine, and valine) because you need them during exercise to maintain muscle tissue, sustain your muscle glycogen supply, and help prevent muscle breakdown. The BCAAs provide up 5 to 10 percent of the calories you burn while training or competing. Note that it is the BCAAs you need to prevent muscle degradation in an endurance event, not whole proteins.

- Water—they all contain it.
- Salt. Salt is added to aid the mineral balance, helping to replace the sodium lost during exercise.
- Chemicals used to retard spoilage. Present in small amounts, these chemicals might include sodium benzoate or potassium sorbate.
- Number of calories. Most gels contain about 100 calories, unless you get one of the new, concentrated versions of the product.

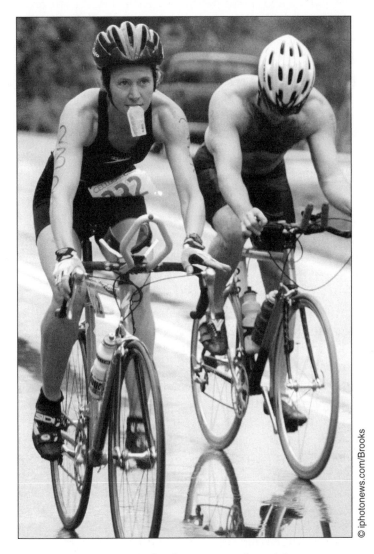

© iphotonews.com/Brooks

Gels offer a sort of energy and the best ones also aid recovery.

• Packaging, which looks a little like the ketchup packs at the ballpark. GU, Clif, and Hammer Nutrition have also introduced multiple-serving packages that you use with a straw. This innovation could be very useful at high altitudes when you need a food that provides quick energy, remains edible in cold temperatures, and doesn't require you to remove your mittens to eat it.

Differences mainly come in the following areas:

• Presence of caffeine.
• Addition of herbs. For example, GU contains chamomile, possibly an anti-inflammatory substance.

You will probably see more performance-related differences between the products in the near future as companies experiment with carbohydrate and herb blends.

Putting the Energy Products in Context

To get a sense of how elite athletes meet energy needs by integrating bars, gels, supplements, meal replacements, and herbal stimulants with whole food during their training and competition, here is a comparison of two diets that are surprisingly similar in one way and very different in another. Wes Hobson, a top Olympic distance and Xterra triathlete, and Bryan Neese, who earned the title "America's Strongest Man" in 1999, have very similar foundation diets: They both emphasize that they really pay attention to the amount of protein they eat daily. They are both keenly aware of how the timing, amount, and quality of their protein and amino acid intake affect their muscle recovery. Where they diverge dramatically is the volume of calories, the use of particular supplements, and the choice of long-term and quick-energy aids (see pages 35-38).

Sometimes the best source of energy makes no scientific sense at all. The psychological boost you get from a fun food can outweigh the nutritional merits of one more energy bar or carbohydrate cocktail. When team Eco-Internet competed in—and later won—the 500-kilometer Eco-Challenge adventure race in British Columbia, their support crew had Domino's drive more than an hour to deliver fresh pizzas to the team when they arrived at a transition area. In the southern Utah Eco-Challenge the year before, my team was pushing hard on day eight, trying to canoe more than 50 miles to the finish line before the race organizers would declare the contest closed. Fatigue and sleep deprivation robbed us of good humor. We just wanted to get there and wondered where we would get the energy to finish. Living on sports foods had become a depressing reality. Seriously hungry as we were, no one had any desire to take even one more bite of an energy bar. At an especially low moment, my teammate, Knute Neihoff, pulled out a treat he had been saving for a time just like this. In my recollection, it was a "hallelujah" occasion that helped restore our energy and our sense of humor: He shared a handful of M&Ms.

Wes Hobson, triathlete   166 pounds

Foundation diet

- Eats animal protein such as meat, poultry, or fish at roughly half his whole-food meals
- Rarely eats sweets, but as a treat, sometimes prepares brownie or cake mix and eats a few scoops (of the mix)
- Balances diet with fruits, vegetables, and whole grains, including bread

Sample training day

Early morning

1 Clif Bar before swim practice; swims 4,000–5,000 yd. (roughly 2.3–2.8 mi., or 3.7–4.6 km); 1,500 yd is intense and the rest is drills

Eats the Clif Bar on the way to the pool—a 15-min. drive—then about 10 min. later, begins swimming. Total elapsed time between eating and training is 25–30 min.

If energy fades during the workout, will eat a Clif Shot ("If I don't have anything to eat before or during the workout, I may make it through, but it's harder for me to recover for a second workout.")

Midmorning

An energy shake consisting of fruit (e.g., a banana or strawberries), Team Pro2 SportFood, Pure Green Power and Pure Red Power ("veggie powders" from Springboard), and water or milk—"I make a full blender so I can have it throughout the day." (total protein from the shake is about 53 gm when made with milk: 37 gm from the meal replacement powder and 16 from the milk)

1 Multivitamin (Team Pro2)

4 tablets Glucosamine Sport Plus (Team Pro2; 1000 mg)

Late morning

During 2–2 1/2-hour group ride, with about 50 min. at his anaerobic threshold

1 Clif Bar

2 Clif Shots

1 water bottle filled with Pro Endurance (Team Pro 2 hydration and recovery drink) "The Clif Bar and Pro Endurance are both for energy, but different types of energy."

Lunch

Turkey sandwich

(continued)

Midafternoon

Nap

Easy 45-min. run (on alternate days, the run is long and involves interval work, but the bike workout lasts only an hour and is relatively easy)

Dinner

Meat, fish, or chicken

Carbohydrates, such as a little bread or potatoes and vegetables

Sample competition day

Olympic-distance triathlon consisting of 1.5-km swim, 40-km bike ride, and 10-km run (1:50 to 2:00 hr.), *or*

Xterra Triathlon consisting of 1.5-km swim, 30-km mountain bike ride, and 10-km run (2:20 to 2:30 hours because the mountain bike portion is more demanding than the Olympic triathlon with a road bike)

Pre-race

1 Clif Bar

1 banana

$\frac{1}{2}$ Clif Bar immediately before the race

Race

2 Clif Shots taped to bike

    1 used 20 min. into the ride

    1 used 20 min. before the end

1 water bottled filled with Pro Endurance

2 Clif Shots during the run

    1 used 10 min. into the run

    1 used 15 min. before the end

"I have a Clif Shot before a water aid station to wash it down."

Bryan Neese, strongman   320 pounds

Foundation diet

- Eats beef at 2 of 3 daily whole-food meals ("I won't eat fish. I won't eat chicken. We have cows in Indiana. We have beef. I'm happy.")
- Rarely eats sweets
- Balances diet with fruits, vegetables, and whole grains, including bread

Sample training day

Early morning

2 scoops Pro Blend 55 (Human Development Technologies) in 12 oz. lowfat milk (total protein in this shake is 67 gm: 55 from the meal replacement powder and 12 from the milk)

2 pancakes or a waffle or bowl of cereal

1 glass orange juice

1 scoop each:

  creatine (5 gm)

  glutamine (5 gm)

6 tablets BCAA (5 gm)

Midmorning

A Pro Blend bar, an apple, or both (total protein from the bar is 32 gm)

Lunch

A couple of servings of whatever they're serving in the cafeteria of the Brownsburg Junior High, where he teaches 7th grade general science; often sandwiches and vegetables

Iced tea

Midafternoon

Pro Blend bar

1 scoop each:

  creatine (5 gm)

  glutamine (5 gm)

6 tablets BCAA (5 gm)

Late afternoon

Weight workout in gym or at home; has access to specialized strongman training equipment primarily through his company, Massive Equipment (on alternate days, he does aerobic training)

3 capsules of Andro Blast (Human Development Technologies), a thermogenic aid containing herbal stimulants; the product also contains Androstenedione, addressed in chapter 4, "Supplementing for Strength."

(continued)

Dinner

1 scoop glutamine (5 gm)

6 tablets BCAA (5 gm)

Beef

Carbohydrates, such as pasta or potatoes and vegetables

Before bed

2 scoops Pro Blend 55 (Human Development Technologies) in 12 oz. lowfat milk, *or*
Pro Blend bar

Sample competition day

12 events conducted over 2 consecutive days, with events separated by about $1/2$ hr. One day's challenges might include events such as:

Farmer's Walk (carrying 2 oxygen cylinders weighing 285 lbs. Each on a 140-yd. course and completing the trek in 90 seconds or less)

Axle Press

Holding 2 SUVs from rolling down a ramp after the brakes are disengaged

Pulling a tour bus

Running with rocks weighing from 230–310 lbs. each, and then placing them on a platform

Super Yoke (getting under a bar that links yokes together, lifting that, and running 120 ft. with 2 tanks weighing a total of 815 lbs)

Pre-competition

Oatmeal and fruit ("as much as I can stomach")

1 scoop each:

    creatine (5 gm)

    glutamine (5 gm)

6 tablets BCAA (5 gm)

Immediately before each contest (six per day)

3–4 capsules of Andro Blast

Lots of water

Do not use this much thermogenic product unless you have extensive experience with it, and are a very large person! Each time Bryan ingests this dosage, he takes in the equivalent of 4 cups of strong coffee, not to mention high dosages of ephedra and hormone. Please see the cautions in chapter 6 in the section on fat burners. "The level (of dosage) I'm taking on competition day is extreme. It is not something good to do every day. . . . I train high school football players and I'd never let any of those guys take it before they play."

A final insight from Bryan on eating for strongman contests: "You'll puke if you eat anything very close to a contest."

CHAPTER 3

Aiding Recovery

Recovery products address the full range of post-workout needs, such as preventing muscle breakdown, feeding muscle growth, replenishing energy, and protecting joints. There is no mistaking a good recovery product, because its effects on your ability to make performance gains show up quickly. Ingesting it at the right time makes it easier to come back from a brutal workout and train hard the next day. Muscle soreness, restless sleep, creaky knees, lack of energy—all the unpleasant conditions you may have come to accept as normal after intense training—don't have to occur at all if you choose your recovery products wisely. To do that, it's important to understand how different types of hard training tax your system and lead to different types of recovery needs.

When you do heavy resistance training (weight training) to make strength gains or to sculpt your body, you create the dual concerns of muscle breakdown and growth. In essence, you break muscle down inside the gym with a brutal workout and then build it outside the gym with proper nutrition and rest. You want to be sure that your recovery products prevent muscle wasting, or continued breakdown of muscle tissue (catabolism), at the same time that they provide anabolic, or muscle building, support. For years, strength and bodybuilding athletes have been aware of the importance of ingesting protein in this process, but it is relatively recent that studies and elite athletes' experiences attest to the powerful effects of minerals such as zinc and magnesium on testosterone production and muscle building. Other substances come into play in recovery as well, such as creatine and essential fatty acids. The effect of heavy weights on your knees, hips, shoulders, and elbows also merits your attention. You can minimize the damage through supplements; you need to weigh the relative advantages of investing in expensive supplements such as glucosamine and chondroitin sulfate to help maintain healthy joints or actually repair cartilage.

If you're an endurance athlete, the long-distance running, biking, swimming, kayaking, and other activities that you do take a lot out of you aerobically and demand a lot from your muscles. You share concerns with strength athletes about preventing muscle breakdown and repairing muscle damage, but you also have workouts and competitions in which glycogen depletion is a reality, loss of fluid—and with it, electrolytes—weakens you, and you have a CO_2 buildup. Your recovery needs are therefore somewhat different. Add to that the effect on your joints of high-impact or repeated motion, and you have additional concerns about protecting your cartilage. The stresses on your body also deplete certain minerals in your body.

And then there are the athletes who train, perhaps for hours at time, doing stunts on bikes, snowboards, or skateboards. There are the gymnasts who do exhausting one-minute routines and divers who might practice stunts on a trampoline, but who spend much of their time between a high board and a deep pool. After periods of explosive action and intense concentration, you need to take care of your muscles just like other athletes; beyond that, there may be other needs as well, depending on your style of training.

Post-Workout Muscle Maintenance: Protein

All sports involve the breakdown of muscle tissue, or catabolism. In trying to make athletic gains, you intensify the process. Instead of doing the same workout everyday, which keeps you at the same level of fitness, you add repetitions or distance to increase your endurance, or weight to increase your strength. Sometimes, in an attempt to step up to a higher performance level, you really shock your body: instead of biking on flat roads, you climb dirt hills; instead of using machines, you rely completely on free weights. To varying degrees, the result is muscle breakdown, possibly even with micro-injuries to the muscle tissue and the accompanying delayed onset muscle soreness (DOMS) that hits a day or two later. Michael Zumpano, founder of Champion Nutrition, offers an engaging explanation of why DOMS occurs. It's useful for understanding more about the formula of products that address the problem:

> When you stress muscle tissue, it leaks out reactive calcium ions. These guys act like tiny buzz saws. Once released from inside the muscle cells, they chew little holes in the cell membranes. White blood cells find these holes and start an inflammatory condition. Ultimately, this causes you to get sore. This sensation of pain is known as delayed onset muscle soreness.

Because certain amino acids—the nitrogen-containing compounds that are the building blocks of protein—are key players in fighting muscle wasting, repairing muscle tissue, and advancing muscle development, you should embrace the benefits of recovery products that deliver them into your bloodstream.

To get the maximum benefit, you want to *ingest a protein/carbohydrate recovery product as soon as possible* after completing a workout. The window of prime opportunity is less than 30 minutes; many experts assert that it is more like 15 minutes. Many recovery products tout the gram-count and quality of their protein without mentioning the carbohydrates included in the formula, but be sure the carbohydrates are there, or add half a ripe banana or some dried fruit to the snack. A combination of protein and carbohydrates outperforms either proteins alone or carbs alone in aiding recovery. Specifically, eating protein with carbohydrates increases the amount of carbs converted and stored in the muscles as

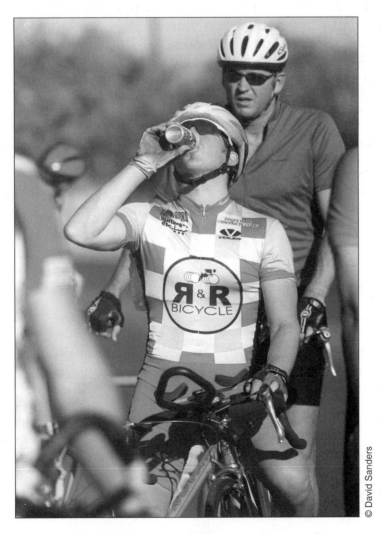

© David Sanders

Consume proteins and carbohydrates within 15 minutes after your workout to maximize recovery.

glycogen. Protein also helps the body repair damaged muscles after exercise and provides the building blocks needed for muscles to grow stronger to handle the stress of future workouts.

Types of Protein

The more complex discussion centers on proteins. Here is where you become familiar with terms such as "isolate," "hydrolyzed," and "concentrate" and with the debates about which protein will serve you best: whey, soy, casein, and so on. Prior to the early 1990s, *whey* was just a nonsense word in a nursery rhyme about some little girl who sat on a tuffet. Strength athletes discussed whether to eat the whole egg or just the white, or how many ounces of chicken breast an athlete should have at one meal. Endurance athletes didn't even give much thought to protein. Many of them were following the *Eat to Win* diet, high in complex carbohydrates and low in fat; their sports food was PowerBar. Suddenly, people like Dr. Scott Connelly, creator of MET-Rx, and three-time Olympian David Jenkins, who developed Designer Protein, began to alert athletes to the role of protein in every athlete's nutritional program. The debate revved up to a sophisticated conversation about isolates, concentrates, and hydrolyzing. For Scott and his early associate, Bill Phillips, who later founded EAS, a focus on the fine points of protein seemed natural—they were both weight-training athletes. As a track and field star, however, David represented a different perspective in the emerging protein powder market, as well as a different formula. Athletes who examined the thinking behind MET-Rx and Designer Protein delved into the question, whey or casein?

The Milk Proteins: Whey and Casein

Marketing battles with scientific overtones complicate the discussion of whey and casein in the world of sports food. To start, in *Contemporary Nutrition: Issues and Insights* (Wardlaw 2000), a glossary entitled "Medical Terminology to Aid in the Study of Nutrition" gives the following definitions for whey and casein:

Whey (WAY)—Proteins, such as lactalbumin, that are found in great amounts in human milk and are easy to digest.

Casein (KAY-seen)—A protein found in milk that forms curds when exposed to acid and is difficult for infants to digest.

Casein is not the same as caseinate, the protein source often found in performance-enhancing products. Caseinates have somewhat different properties from casein.

Before you take a closer look at casein and whey, consider that the commercial source of both of them—cow's milk—is between 20 and 40 percent protein, with skim milk having a higher protein content than whole milk. The carbohydrate percentage of cow's milk ranges from 30 for whole up to 55 percent for skim. Of course, the total calories for an eight-ounce glass of whole milk is nearly double that of skim, and the difference is fat.

Casein accounts for about 80 percent of the protein in cow's milk. Casein products are manufactured from skim milk, but the processes differ slightly depending on what kind of casein is being made. The casein that ends up as caseinates is lactic acid casein. Neutralizing the acid casein with some kind of salt makes a caseinate like sodium caseinate, calcium caseinate, or potassium caseinate. The product you'll find most in performance-enhancing foods is calcium caseinate.

Calcium caseinate has the following characteristics:

- It's soluble in water.
- It's high in glutamine, an important amino acid that supports lean muscle mass.
- It is more slowly digested than the whey or soy protein sources found in food designed for athletes.
- Technically speaking, it is lactose free, but that doesn't mean that a person with protein allergies won't react to it. It also doesn't mean that it's nondairy in a strict kosher or vegan sense.

Sweet dairy whey is a watery byproduct of cheese making. It's skimmed off after the process uses up the casein molecules. Until the early 1980s, manufacturers poured it out, fed it to pigs, or let it run off into fields, where it served as a foul-smelling fertilizer. During the 1980s, manufacturers began experimenting with whey filtration to separate the proteins from the water. Among the results are the following forms of whey, now used in performance-enhancing foods:

- **Whey protein concentrate** is sweet dairy whey that has been concentrated to get more protein per unit. The process gets rid of some of the nonprotein materials such as ash, carbohydrates, fat, and lactose. It doesn't get rid of all of them, however, and the amount of protein in the remaining concentrate can range quite a bit. Although some companies undoubtedly use cheaper, less concentrated forms, the standard for a whey protein concentrate is about 70 to 80 percent protein.

(continued)

• Whey protein can be concentrated even more to produce **whey protein isolate**, which has even less fat, carbohydrates, and other extraneous components than the concentrate form. Whey isolates should be 80 to 90 percent protein.

• **Hydrolyzed protein** has been bathed to break down amino acids. In effect, the hydrolysis process breaks down the protein structure, making smaller protein chains available. Hydrolyzed whey is easily absorbed—which is potentially good in the sense that the body can use the amino acids quickly—but it has less desirable characteristics, too. For one thing, it tastes awful: the hydrolysis yields an extremely bitter product.

The characteristics of whey proteins change somewhat depending on the form, but all whey proteins share certain general traits:

• They are complete proteins; that is, they have all the essential amino acids. They have an especially high ratio of branched chain amino acids (BCAAs), consisting of leucine, isoleucine, and valine. (The BCAAs are important for muscle building, and a deficiency in one of them will cause muscle loss. Unlike other amino acids, BCAAs are metabolized in the muscle rather than the liver.

• They are absorbed in the system very quickly; in fact, they don't even sit in the stomach waiting to be broken down: they go straight to the lower intestine.

• They stimulate the immune system.

Much of the whey-versus-casein debate is really an issue of timing. Because a caseinate enters the system relatively slowly, it has more value in a meal replacement taken before bedtime or in the hours before a workout than it does in the minutes after a workout, when you want amino acids racing through your body. Whey's quick absorption makes it an extremely desirable recovery aid in that immediate post-workout period, as well as a good protein pump first thing in the morning.

David Jenkins's emergence as a major player in the protein debates followed a long, slow process of learning about supplements and nutrition throughout the late 1970s and early 1980s. It roughly paralleled the early research on whey.

David won a silver medal in the 4 × 400 meter relay in the 1972 Munich Games using a fairly standard eating program and no help from chemicals. But three years later, after recapturing the world's attention as the fastest 400-meter runner, he started exploring performance-enhancing options. He says that during the time he prepared for the 1976 and 1980 Olympics and participated in them, "I was exposed to everything from quackery to hard-core sports drugs." He started using anabolic steroids periodically.

Having already earned a chemical engineering degree from Edinburgh University, he undertook postgraduate work in business administration and was awarded a Winston Churchill Traveling Fellowship. As part of his study of recreational facilities in the United States, he trained at the University of California, Los Angeles (UCLA). There he ran into the 1966 world record holder in decathlon, Russ Hodge, who introduced him to a high-protein shake and high-potency vitamins and minerals. David used the products while he tried to recover from an injury and marveled at how they seemed to help him. During the same period, he roomed with the team doctor for the Southern California Striders and discovered lean California eating—salads, fresh vegetables, chicken breasts, and fish. It was nothing like the heavy foods that had retained popularity in his native Great Britain. Although David looks at this time as a turning point in his understanding of how nutrition aids performance, he adds a caveat: "Of course, it was difficult to be totally objective about it because of the steroid overlay."

In his subsequent effort to study all aspects of performance enhance-ment in sport, David exploited his international renown and collected the nutritional wisdom and anecdotes of fellow world-class athletes. He looked at the rainbow of substances "from food to fool's gold." In the midst of this process, the U.S. government paid him a dubious compli-ment, crediting him for 70 percent of the anabolic steroid traffic in the country, and briefly gave him room and board in a federal prison. It was an end and a beginning.

After the experience, David started a company "devoid of all of this," with a straight and narrow focus on macronutrients and with particular research into high-quality protein. A couple of years later he was going head to head with people like Scott Connelly and Bill Phillips.

Protein's Role in Recovery

The development of competing protein-product formulas reflects some conflicting thoughts about the relative merits of different product sources. From the early days, David Jenkins has carried the torch for whey. In the opposing camps are the casein advocates, the soy advocates, and those who advocate mixing several sources together. The champions of these different protein sources aren't literally inherent adversaries, of course, but they do oppose one another in their marketing efforts, which attempt to persuade consumers that one way is the best. Despite this disagreement on sources, most of the competitors concur on two other issues when it comes to protein's role in recovery:

1.   When you add carbohydrates to a protein delivery system, you increase the insulin release. The insulin helps drive the nutrients into action. In essence, the carbohydrates help shuttle nutrients at an accelerated rate for growth and recovery.

2.   Timing is key. The initial window of opportunity is less than a half hour after your workout. The exercise creates chemical reactions in your muscles that, combined with the insulin, immediately put nutrients to work for your recovery. If you get the right formula into your body on time, you support muscle growth, prevention of muscle wasting, lactic acid removal, and much more.

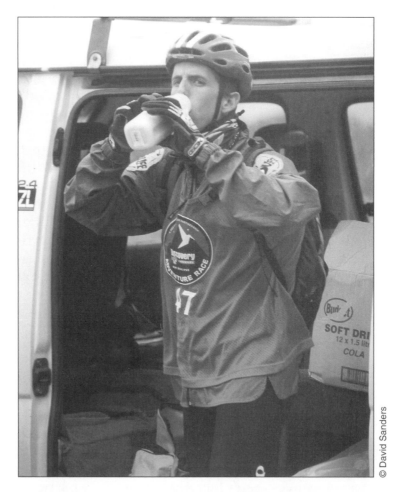

© David Sanders

Manufacturers advocate different protein sources than others. Take this into account when deciding if a product is right for you.

Throughout much of this book, you are encouraged to read labels and to assess the formulas of products so that you can match your individual needs. When you evaluate post-workout protein products, however, you'll want to become more familiar with the companies behind the products. In some cases, the labels on products disclose only partial ingredient information or use unconventional terms, and you can't count on a federal regulatory body to discipline sports-food companies right now (at least, not in the United States) unless they make medical claims. In other cases, companies genuinely do use unique formulas or processes; therefore, they may include terms on the label that you've never seen before.

For example, MET-Rx calls its protein blend METAMYOSYN and EAS calls its blend MyoPro. Another example concerns the dairy company now called Davisco, which purchased patents to use a processing method called "ultrafiltration" to make a high-quality whey protein called Bipro. A third example of unconventional terminology is "microfraction selection technology cross flow quadrafiltration manufacturing process." Reading the label tells you nothing about what this process entails. In contrast, other companies provide detailed descriptions of such terms; unfortunately, the descriptions themselves sound like gibberish to most athletes. The message here is, don't assume that highfalutin terms reflect sound science.

For a prime example of how companies may mislead you by offering only partial information, consider the reporting of fat content. Bodybuilders in particular often obsess on the amount of fat in a product and compare performance-enhancing foods primarily on the basis of how much fat is supposedly in them. What are you supposed to think when you evaluate a product label that highlights whey protein with no fat or cholesterol next to another that lists whey protein and some of those other components? All whey proteins, which are derived from milk, contain some amount of fat and cholesterol. The more the whey protein is processed to increase the percentage of protein and reduce the amount of nonprotein components, the less fat and cholesterol remain. It may be just 2 percent of the total product, but it's still there. The only thing that can make the fat "disappear" is misleading labeling and deceptive ad copy.

Another common example of misleading labeling concerns glycerine. Glycerine may have some value to athletes in terms of fluid retention. In terms of marketing functions, however, its value is clear: Glycerine improves the texture of high-protein bars, and including it boosts the total calories of a bar without adding grams of carbohydrates. You will often find that this component is simply hidden among the ingredients of protein bars. The macronutrient list might indicate a total of 260 calories, with 30 grams of protein, 6 carbohydrate grams, and 5 grams of fat. Add that up: 30 grams $\times$ 4 = 120 calories; 6 grams $\times$ 4 = 24 calories; 5 grams $\times$ 9 = 45 calories. The total is 189. What is the source of the other 71 calories, or nearly 30 percent of the total calories? Glycerine. Check the list of ingredients; it will be among the first.

Manufacturers most often tie the pitch on their labels to types of protein—whey, casein, egg albumin, soy, or some "patented formula"—and to the method of processing the protein, such as "hydrolyzed," "micro-filtered," or some "patented approach." As indicated previously, claims of patented formulas and patented protein-processing methods can be valid, but those phrases do not equate to promises of high performance.

Unfortunately, the number of confusing terms in the ingredients list sometimes seems to relate directly to the drama and persuasion in the advertising copy. Many manufacturers seem determined to make you feel like a student in a college chemistry class, perhaps to humble you so that you are more vulnerable to their hype. They throw every "micro" this and "ultra" that into the stew of descriptions until you feel just stupid enough to think the manufacturer knows it all.

Your choice of product may depend on some simple considerations such as how the product tastes, whether or not it gives you gas, whether or not you feel hungry after you take it, and so on. A more scientific way of approaching these considerations might be expressed in terms of the following:

- Quality as determined by the amino acids the product contains
- Quality as measured by protein efficiency ratio (PER), biological value (BV), or net protein utilization (NPU)
- Digestibility
- Post-workout contribution to muscle-building (anabolism)
- Post-workout protection against muscle breakdown (catabolism)

What can algae do that athletes can't? Algae can synthesize all the amino acids it needs to live—the same amino acids that humans need, but people can synthesize only some of them (Stryer 1995). Amino acids are the component parts of proteins. You need all 22 amino acids for the health and growth of living tissues, but you must obtain nine of them—the "essential" amino acids—either by eating foods that contain them or by combining foods that together enable you to synthesize them. Animal products—meat, fish, poultry, eggs, and dairy products—give you the essential amino acids. Examples of nonanimal foods that combine to give you what you need are rice and beans and peanut butter on whole-wheat bread (grains and legumes), rice and sesame seeds (grains and seeds), sesame seeds and peanuts (seeds and legumes), creamy pea soup (milk product and legumes), and macaroni and cheese (milk product and grains) (Lappe 1976; Gershoff 1996). The only nonanimal food that delivers all essential amino acids on its own is soybeans.

Knowing these fundamentals about amino acids, you can see why performance-enhancing foods designed for recovery feature some form of egg protein, whey, casein, soy, rice, or some combination of those ingredients. The reasoning takes shape even more when you know that these are highly digestible forms of protein, especially when they've been subjected to certain types of processing. They enter your system and then break down into the amino acids that you need to avert muscle breakdown and to help build muscle tissue. A steak or fish sticks wouldn't have nearly the same post-workout recovery effect, because your body has to work much harder to break down the dietary protein into the component parts it needs on the cellular level.

A brief look at the protein efficiency ratio (PER), biological value (BV), or net protein utilization (NPU) will clear up key misconceptions about the claims recovery products make about proteins and will set the stage for evaluating those products.

Some scientists question the value of the PER, because it's based on studies involving animals only. All of the quality-measurement studies referenced here, however, can be (and are) done with animals. Many nutrition authorities who focus on athletes' needs stand by PER, because it measures how efficiently a protein stimulates muscle growth. Other scientists question the value of BV, because BV testing is done with subjects who are fasting, which alters certain body processes. Those who defend BV argue that it measures how digestible protein is and how efficiently the body uses it. If a food has a high BV, a relatively high proportion of the protein in the food is retained in the body. Franco Columbu, a former Mr. Olympia and a doctor of chiropractic with a PhD in nutrition, is among those who prefer to rate foods according to the NPU. Similar to BV, NPU is yet another way of describing the rate of protein absorption into the bloodstream.

PER measurements of the proteins you see in performance-enhancing foods generally range from around 1.8 (soy) to 3.5 (egg whites). The total range is 0 to 3.5, with the standard being 2.5 for casein, which is the major milk protein. Researchers determine PER by feeding rats for 28 days and measuring their weight gain.

PER = amount of weight gained ÷ amount of protein consumed

Based on PER alone, if you aren't allergic to egg whites, or albumen, you would choose a recovery product that includes egg protein if your aim is building muscle. The argument doesn't stop there, though. Many companies flaunt the high PERs of their whey protein products, claiming they are nearly as high as (or higher than) the PER of egg protein. Depending on the manufacturing methods used to process the whey, the claims may be legitimate. If you are a bodybuilder or strength athlete, these nuances are important. If you are an endurance athlete, you don't have to be as concerned about the number because your focus is more on preventing muscle breakdown after a hard workout than on building muscle.

BV and NPU are similar in that they are both determined by measuring nitrogen uptake versus the amount of nitrogen that is excreted. In other words, they measure how much nitrogen the body retains, which relates directly to how much protein the body retains.

- Who cares about retaining nitrogen?
  - As an athlete, you do, because it relates to the condition of your muscle tissue.
- Why do you need protein to get that nitrogen?
  - Unlike the other nutrients, which are composed only of carbon, hydrogen, and oxygen, protein includes nitrogen and sulfur.

BV ratings are generally expressed as whole numbers, with ratings for various foods determined by how they compare to egg whites, which are arbitrarily assigned a BV of 100. The BV ratings for the proteins most often discussed as ingredients in recovery products—some form of soy, milk proteins, and egg—range from about 74 for soy to 159 for high-quality whey. Beef has a BV of 80. The NPU ratings only go to 100 and are expressed as percentages; for example, eggs earn a rating of 88 percent and soybeans a rating of 48 percent.

It would be wrong to assume that the relatively lower numbers assigned to soybeans or soy products in all these evaluation systems make it a "bad" protein for athletes—not so! First of all, it's important to put soy into context with other proteins. For example, the approximate BV of rice is 59, and that of beans is 49, as compared to soy's 74. In addition, research indicates that soy protein is easily digested; that it is the only vegetable source of all essential amino acids (that is, it has a high-quality amino acid profile); that it has cancer-fighting benefits; that it may work to speed up the metabolism; and that it has myriad other potential benefits, including raising the level of testosterone. These qualities make soy valuable to all types of athletes, but they do not necessarily make it the main protein you want in a recovery product.

Advertising copy sometimes refers to PER or BV in a misleading way. For example, one company claims that it chose whey protein isolate for its nutrition bar because whey has more than double the BV of caseinate or soy protein. That statement may be theoretically true, but you have no way of knowing whether or not the company actually used high-quality whey protein isolate. The BV in this case is a gimmick, not a useful piece of information.

Another misleading ploy in advertising material concerns the interpretation of studies, which may or may not even include references to measurements such as PER or BV. A famous study (Boirie et al. 1997) at the Université Clermont in Auvergne, France, has fueled the assertion that whey quickly boosts amino acids in the blood and that it is therefore the single most useful protein in building muscle after a workout. The same study has bolstered the claim that casein is the one and only protein to prevent muscle breakdown.

The study concludes that "the speed of protein digestion and amino acid absorption from the gut has a major effect on whole body protein anabolism after one single meal" and that whey is the undisputed winner when it comes to rate of absorption. It also states, however, that with casein, "plasma amino acid concentrations are lower, resulting in a lower oxidation and in a lesser increase of protein synthesis, but also in an inhibition of protein breakdown." Don't rush, therefore, to judge one protein as "the one and only one" you will need at every time of day and in every circumstance.

Protein Recovery Products: An Overview

Animal Proteins

- **Milk protein, or complete milk protein,** is protein from cow's milk that has gone through a filtration process; the casein and whey are still together. You may realize increased benefits with a protein like whey, which acts more quickly.
- **Casein/caseinates** prevent muscle breakdown. It is absorbed more slowly than its sister milk protein, whey.
- **Whey** builds muscles. It is absorbed more quickly than casein.
- **Egg protein** has very high ratings in terms of protein efficiency and support for building muscle. It contains the highest quantities of some key amino acids, namely, valine, alanine, methionine, and phenylalanine. Unfortunately, allergies related to egg white, or albumin, are not uncommon; phenylketonurics (people with this allergy) are specifically sensitive to phenylalanine and should look for warnings about its presence in the product formula.

(continued)

Vegetable Proteins

- **Soy protein isolate** can contain more than 90 percent protein and provides a high amount of glutamine, arginine, and branched chain amino acids. A bonus advantage is that soy isolates, which lower cholesterol levels, can increase your production of thyroid-stimulating hormone and thyroxin, both of which can boost your ability to burn fat.
- **Rice protein** is relatively high in glutamine and alanine. The former amino acid plays an important role in preventing muscle breakdown, and the latter is the key carrier of nitrogen to the muscle.

Carbohydrates

A high-glycemic carbohydrate should be part of your protein recovery product. If your preferred protein powder or premixed drink does not include it, add it yourself. Enjoy your drink with a banana or a couple of rice cakes to make sure you replenish your glycogen stores.

The main forms of protein-focused recovery products are powders that can be blended or shaken with liquid into a drink, pre-blended protein drinks, and protein bars, which don't have the same digestibility (hence, performance) advantages as their drinkable counterparts. In fact, bars are sort of a last-resort recovery product; top strength and endurance athletes rely on drinks. Convenience is a legitimate issue even for some elite athletes, but as the audience for recovery products grows, manufacturers will undoubtedly find more convenient ways of packaging high-quality protein formulas.

Ironman Triathlon champion Peter Reid remembers that it took him years to discover that he needed a recovery product, and then, when he finally did, he used the product only sporadically because he hated the thought of cleaning the blender.

For several years before his rise to the top, Peter struggled with nutritional habits and products that did not serve him well. When he was a cyclist in high school, his coach made everyone on the team abide by Robert Haas's *Eat to Win*, a 1983 book that recommends a diet high in complex carbohydrates and low in fat and protein. Peter stuck with that program for years. "I was eating all the time," he says. "Tons of pasta, tons of bagels—never putting a conscious effort on eating protein." The Canadian remembers going to big races in the States and thinking, "I'm the fattest guy on the starting line." That certainly didn't give him any advantages.

Finally, in 1995, while lying on a massage table in southern California, Peter got his first glimpse of a tub of protein powder. He asked the massage therapist if he was on diet. The therapist was incredulous: "You never make a recovery drink after training? Oh, Peter!" He then passed along a "trade secret" from another of his clients, John Tomac, one of the biggest stars of mountain biking in the eighties and early nineties. Immediately after that, Peter began incorporating protein shakes into his recovery regimen. He noticed that he wasn't as hungry as he used to be for a large meal after intense training and that he was bouncing back a little more quickly. "There's something to this," he concluded, and he began doing recovery shakes after hard workouts—except when he didn't feel like dealing with the blender.

Peter needed something that could help him become more consistent about using a protein-focused recovery product. In 1998, his wife, Ironman triathlon champion Lori Bowden, introduced him to a protein formula in a tube. The product, JogMate from Pharmavite, was a water-based pudding that Lori simply squirted in her mouth after a hard workout. Peter says, "It was so easy. You walked in the house. There was a tube. It was a no-brainer."

Their story highlights one of the fundamental reasons you, as an active person, probably choose one product over another—convenience. If you do a hard workout and then have to rush off to an office or classroom, you want the best of all worlds in a recovery product: the right ratio of essential amino acids and carbs in a easily digestible product that you can carry around. Alternatively, you may want a product that dissolves easily in water: something you can throw in a cup, take to the water cooler, swish around, and drink. Read the instructions on the can and look for the directive, "stir," rather than "mix in a blender."

Remember one final note about protein recovery powders: After you mix the drink, consume it immediately to get the maximum benefit. Don't let it sit around while you compare notes with your gym buddies.

Recovery After Hard Cardio: Carbohydrates, Electrolytes, and Water

Recommendations on protein recovery products emphasize the importance of high-glycemic carbohydrates. Don't forget that carbohydrates help make the most of the protein you ingest to aid recovery. Also note that protein affects the rate of absorption of carbohydrates you consume to aid your recovery after an endurance workout.

Protein's main job may be to help you build and maintain muscles, but you need carbohydrates to fuel them. If you've been running, cycling, or doing any intense cardiorespiratory exercise for more than an hour with your heart working at 60 to 80 percent of maximum, then your liver and muscle glycogen levels might be very low. During the sustained activity,

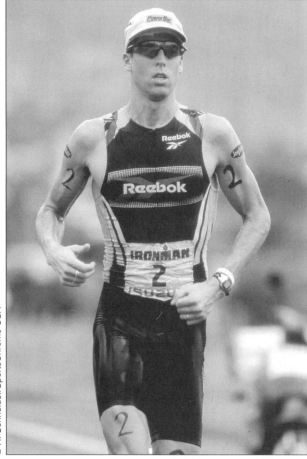

© H. Schneider/SportsChrome USA

Peter Reid reaped the benefits when he made his recovery routine more consistent.

as well as in the hour or two after the activity, a product that helps bring your glycogen levels up can serve you well. You also lose water and sodium during endurance activities, particularly if you do them in the heat, and you affect the balance of your other electrolytes: potassium, calcium, magnesium, and chloride.

There are two ways to address glycogen depletion, dehydration, and electrolyte imbalance with performance-enhancing products: a specially formulated drink or a combination of water and a sports food. The first thing to note is that drinking something is always part of the process. Figure 3.1 highlights the importance by illustrating how dramatically performance diminishes with fluid loss.

If you use a sports drink during an event to aid recovery as you go, be sure it has a low carbohydrate concentration (around 6 percent). Ideally, it should have 14 to 19 grams of carbs per eight-ounce serving—6 to 8 percent. Anything with a carbohydrate concentration greater than 10 percent can be used as part of a carbohydrate loading program, but you

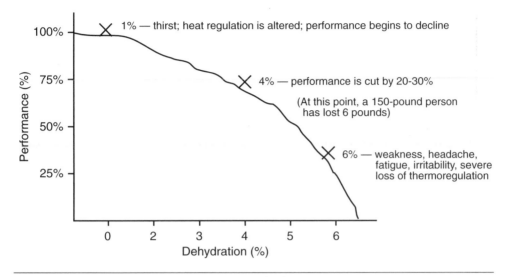

Figure 3.1 Performance diminishes with dehydration.

want to stay away from high-carb products around race time, because they can cause diarrhea, nausea, or cramping. On the other end of the spectrum, a drink with a concentration of 5 percent or less won't give you the boost you want.

Follow these broad guidelines on what to look for in sports drinks products and what to stay away from. First, don't choose a drink that's carbonated, contains a stimulant, or is full of refined sugar, like a cola drink or one of the clear, bubbly beverages that gives you a jolt from either caffeine or herbs. Second, remember that water alone isn't enough to support your full recovery after an endurance workout or competition. These insights are based on research and on the experience of elite athletes interviewed for this book.

One piece of research (Brouns, Hawley, and Jeukendrup 1998) studied the effects of different rehydration drinks on competitive cyclists. After their workouts, some of the cyclists were given caffeinated soft drinks, others low-sodium mineral water, and others a carbohydrate-electrolyte solution—a sports drink. The athletes who drank the soft drinks and the mineral water showed a marked loss of every one of the electrolytes. Moreover, the athletes who consumed the soft drinks were at a further disadvantage, because the caffeine provoked urination; essentially, it dehydrated them even more. (Other stimulants, such as ephedra, have the same effect.) In contrast, the athletes who ingested the sports drinks were able to rehydrate and boost their sodium, magnesium, and calcium levels. The drink did not affect their potassium and chloride levels, however. (That deficit will be addressed separately.) The study concluded that drinking water or soda with caffeine after a workout results in a negative electrolyte balance. Consuming a carbohydrate-electrolyte drink with moderate amounts of sodium, magnesium, and calcium definitely helps an athlete recover.

Regarding the carbonation issue, consider that part of your body's natural process of producing energy relies on the oxygen (O_2) you breathe. A byproduct of the process is carbon dioxide (CO_2). You don't want a lot of carbon dioxide in your system because it's poisonous to cells. It's important to eliminate the excess, which you generally do through normal cardiovascular processes (blood flow and heart action) and respiratory processes (breathing). Endurance athletes, such as marathon runners, however, demand more than normal functioning from the body. When you push hard aerobically for an extended period of time, you tax your body's ability to eliminate excess carbon dioxide, and you face a potential CO_2 buildup. As your body works to eliminate the extra CO_2, don't choose a recovery drink that's carbonated—that is, a beverage made bubbly by the infusion of CO_2 gas. Ironically, you will sometimes see beverage companies offering bubbly drinks during and after races. At the very least, dilute any carbonated beverage by adding an equal amount of water before your drink it. Otherwise, beware of the most obvious negative reaction: carbonation can cause stomach bloating. In short, you may feel lousy in addition to the beverage not providing the benefits you seek.

Carbohydrate recovery drinks include these options:

- Powders you mix with water; the amount can be easily adjusted depending on your taste and on whether you consume the drink during or after the event
- Premixed drinks with a prescribed concentration of carbohydrates and other nutrients and additives; in terms of both composition and packaging, these drinks are usually better suited for use after workouts

There are other ways to view your drink options, too, particularly in light of the electrolyte discussion. They concern sodium, calcium, and other elements in the drink; herbs for different aspects of recovery; and patented (or patent-pending) formulas that distinguish one carbohydrate mix from another.

Research (Maughan and Shirreffs 1998) has shown that electrolyte loss is a personal matter. The optimum drink for you may be quite different from that of another athlete. This fact is one reason why some top trainers persistently believe that athletes don't lose enough electrolytes in the first 90 minutes of intense aerobic exercise to require any recovery fluid except water. At the same time, there is widespread agreement that ingesting either carbohydrate drinks or water and a carbohydrate bar, for example, replenishes lost glycogen. The electrolyte research cited previously reflects current thinking that replenishing some of the electrolytes is not only desirable but also necessary for endurance athletes. Your individual metabolism, temperature, and level of exertion all influence the electrolyte loss, however, so the same drink with the same concentration of carbs and electrolytes won't be ideal for every athlete or even for the same athlete under different conditions.

This variability is one of many reasons you should keep a log to help you refine your workout regimen and your choices of sports food. Pay attention to how you feel after a brutal cardiorespiratory workout, and adjust the amount of fluid you take in according to how you feel. Signs of electrolyte imbalance include fatigue, tremors, diarrhea, and nausea.

The following are electrolytes:

- Sodium
- Potassium
- Calcium
- Magnesium
- Chloride

Generally speaking—and this is just a benchmark number—a good sodium level for a recovery drink is 100 to 110 milligrams for every eight ounces. Take a look at what's out there: the sodium (Na) content in sports drinks ranges from around 10 milligrams to well over 100.

Research indicates that you don't sweat out vitamins, so even though you should take vitamins to support your athletic goals, your recovery drink doesn't need to include them.

Mineral Rights and Wrongs

Your athletic performance will be adversely affected if you have a deficiency of certain minerals and trace elements. This problem is a recovery issue, because athletes often suffer mineral deficiencies as a direct result of exercise. There are two reasons: intense activity increases the metabolic need for minerals, and athletes tend to excrete excessive amounts of minerals. Studies by the U.S. Food and Drug Administration have documented that the concentration of minerals such as magnesium and potassium in the urine of athletes on a workout day can be nearly double that of a non-workout day. Minerals move out of the body with sweat, too, so exercising in a hot climate can make the problem considerably worse.

If you compound this mineral loss through sports with factors that cause deficiencies in the general population, the effect on athletic performance can be profound. Two big examples of substances that exacerbate the problem are birth control pills and some deodorants. Birth control pills can cause elevated copper levels, and an excess of copper means reduced levels of zinc. Zinc has several key functions in the body—from promoting active taste buds to maintaining a strong immune system—but the roles most important to athletes are its abilities to break down and utilize carbohydrates and to build muscle. As for deodorants, those with aluminum sap the body of magnesium. BALCO Laboratories in Burlingame, California, did a mineral depletion study with the Seattle Supersonics and found that 80 percent of the basketball team had seriously low magnesium levels. Victor Conte, who conducted the study, discovered the dominant problem: The players used antiperspirants with aluminum chlorohydrate. Aluminum inhibits the body's ability to absorb and use magnesium. The same problem can occur in areas of the United States where hard water is treated with sodium aluminate to prevent calcium and magnesium deposits from building up in water pipes. The most noticeable effects of mineral deficiencies in athletes are shown in table 3.1.

If you notice muscle weakness, poor night vision, stress fractures, slow-healing wounds, cramps, sleeplessness, or other chronic problems even though you eat a diet that supports your athletic goals and you take a multivitamin, then you have reason to suspect a deficiency in vital minerals and trace elements.

The trace mineral vanadium may also be very useful to athletes in the form of vanadyl sulfate. This substance is under investigation but there is no conclusive evidence at this time. Studies are exploring its possible role in helping blood glucose enter muscle cells, a function similar to insulin's; it may increase insulin sensitivity in muscle cells only and not in fat cells. If that hypothesis is true, then vanadyl sulfate can truly aid bodybuilders by storing glucose in muscles and leaving less to be ultimately stored as fat. The effect would be greater muscle fullness—the sometimes-elusive "pump." If you take it, remember that it's an experi-

Table 3.1 Mineral Deficiencies

Deficiency	Result
Zinc	Decrease in muscle strength and endurance
Magnesium	Decrease of oxygen transport to muscle tissue
Chromium	Depressed energy metabolism
Copper	Weakened connective tissue, ligaments, and tendons
Iron	Decrease of oxygen transport throughout the body

ment and, as with any experiment, you should not exceed manufacturer's recommended dosages and stop taking it after a few weeks to evaluate the effects.

Because many athletes are growing more aware of their need for micronutrients, such as minerals, supplement manufacturers are rushing to meet the need. The result is sometimes a product stuffed with minerals that doesn't work harmoniously if ingested at the same time. For example, the label of one protein product declares that it offers zinc and magnesium in a trademarked combination along with a hefty dose of calcium. Calcium inhibits magnesium and zinc absorption. This product is an example of overkill. Beware of products with labels that promise all the protein, minerals, and vitamins you need in one serving. To avoid wasting your money, know when to ingest certain foods and supplements, and know how much you need.

When you begin to address your deficiency by experimenting with supplements—and it will be an experiment in the beginning—use the chart in table 3.2 as a guide to pairing minerals and taking them at appropriate times. Also, carefully document how you feel and what kind of changes you notice. On the positive side, more restful sleep and even more entertaining dreams can be an immediate result of zinc-magnesium supplementation at bedtime. On the negative side, excess magnesium can cause diarrhea and too much zinc can impair the function of white blood cells and lower good (HDL) cholesterol. The upper limit of magnesium for an athlete training hard is about 800 mg/day and about 60 mg/day for zinc.

Your nutrition log will help you to refine your new program, ultimately hastening the impact on your performance and saving you money: You don't want to buy supplements that do little or nothing to change how you feel. As you invest in mineral supplements, remember that all athletes don't have the same requirements. The type of exercise you do, your level of exertion, and the food you eat are three key factors that influence your need for supplementation.

The best way to determine whether or not you have a mineral or trace element deficiency is to go through blood and urine tests. BALCO Laboratories uses a machine called the inductively coupled plasma (ICP) atomic emission spectrometer. It ascertains the precise trace mineral status of athletes, including Olympic swimming and track and field athletes, the Miami Dolphins, tennis star Michael Chang, and dozens of the world's top professional bodybuilders. The ICP spectrometer analyzes a sample for essential minerals, trace elements, and toxic metals, such as lead and aluminum.

Even before BALCO conducts an analysis, however, athletes complete a comprehensive health questionnaire. You should do the same at the

Table 3.2 The Mineral Chart

Mineral or trace element	Function(s)	Cause(s) of deficiency in athletes	Absorption increased by:	Absorption decreased by:	When and how much/comments (averages—individual needs vary)
Calcium	Builds bones and strength	Vegetarian diet; high-protein diet can cause more calcium excretion	Vitamins A and D; stomach acids	Magnesium	1,200 mg/day; hard exercise is linked to calcium retention, so that supplementation may be unnecessary; if taken, choose calcium carbonate, not antacids with calcium
Chromium	Aids insulin in regulating glucose and fat metabolism	Hard exercise and stress	Amino acid chelates	Zinc, iron, and magnesium	100–200 mg/day between breakfast and lunch; take with copper
Copper	Supports strong connective tissue; synthesizes *hemoglobin* (main part of red blood cells; key to energy production)	Hard exercise and stress	Amino acids	Calcium, iron, zinc, molybdenum, and vitamin C	2–4 mg/day between breakfast and lunch; take with chromium
Iron	Feeds hemoglobin (see above) and *myglobin* (transfers oxygen to muscle cells)	Hard exercise and stress	Vitamin C	Calcium, magnesium, zinc, copper, chromium, and manganese; caffeinated beverages	15–25 mg/day between lunch and dinner; take with selenium; needs can vary widely; best sources are animal products—red meat, chicken, and tuna

Magnesium	Plays a key role in muscle and nerve functioning; aids tissue repair and muscle growth	Hard exercise and stress	Vitamin D	Calcium and sodium	400–500 mg/day before bedtime; take with zinc
Manganese	Supports protein and energy metabolism	Deficiencies are unlikely, but could be diet-related		Calcium and iron	Supplementation shouldn't be necessary; good sources are whole grains and legumes
Potassium	Acts with sodium and chloride to maintain balance in body fluids	Loss of body fluid, as during an endurance race		Calcium and magnesium	Follow guidelines on using an electrolyte replacement drink during and after intense exercise
Selenium	Supports proper heart functioning; protects against toxic doses of some heavy metals	Deficiencies are unlikely, but could be diet-related	Amino acids	Copper	Supplementation shouldn't be necessary and probably isn't desirable; too much can cause skin problems and cavities
Sodium	Acts with potassium and chloride to maintain balance in body fluids	Loss of body fluid, as during an endurance race; the body can't store sodium, so it must be consumed	Amino acids	Calcium and magnesium	Need 200 mg a day, which should come easily with food. Follow guidelines on using an electrolyte replacement drink during and after intense exercise
Zinc	Aids in breakdown and use of carbs and in protein synthesis	Hard exercise and stress; could also be caused by a vegetarian diet	Amino acids	Calcium, iron, manganese, selenium, copper; whole-grain foods and soy foods	20–30 mg/day before bedtime; take with magnesium

Data courtesy of Bay Area Laboratory Co-Operative, Burlingame, California.

start of your program. A questionnaire like the one included as the appendix of this book can help raise your awareness of your symptoms and can point to possible non-sport causes of nutrient deficiencies. You can also come back to it after a month of supplementation and see if your answers have changed. As a corollary, it's a valuable source of information if you decide to visit a testing organization like BALCO, a nutritionist, or a doctor to seek professional guidance.

When Victor Conte launched BALCO and began testing athletes in the mid-1980s, he first looked at caloric intake to see how athletes could make up their deficiencies through diet. He found that approach was not reasonable. The athletes needed to bring up their levels quickly and sustain them, but food alone would not do the job, partially because so many antagonistic relationships exist between the minerals (for example, the zinc-blocking ability of calcium). As a consequence, Victor sent the athletes to a local health food store to buy mineral supplements when he detected deficiencies. He was surprised when they returned for retesting and still showed low levels. The experience drove him to look more closely at the forms of minerals the athletes took—oxides, citrates, and aspartates—and at the time of day they took their supplements. His own products, such as the ZMA formula licensed to several companies, focus on aspartates.

Joint Aids: Not Just for Retired Quarterbacks

You expect someone like Joe Montana to get on the radio and talk about the pain of osteoarthritis. Creaky joints seem like the natural outcome of a couple of decades of pounding on the football field. Although the kind of joint overuse and abuse that a professional football player experiences may in fact provoke osteoarthritis, there is also a theory that a chemical imbalance causes the condition and that the wear-and-tear of sports only makes it considerably worse. Combined with an imbalance, lots of tennis, heavy weightlifting, hard running, or other stressful and repetitive actions may accelerate the breakdown of cartilage, the cushioning for your bones.

This theory could explain why the signs of osteoarthritis sometimes appear during the peak of an athlete's career. You can be in your 30s and have to lean heavily on the railing as you descend the stairs from the gym after a workout. You don't have to be a wrinkled old woman to rub your sore elbow after an hour on the tennis court. On a long run day, even a world-class marathoner in her early 40s might wish Mother Nature had designed knees and hips differently.

Many athletes rely solely on nonsteroidal anti-inflammatory drugs (NSAIDs) to subdue these aches. Without question, NSAIDs like naproxen, ibuprofen, and aspirin are useful; they relieve pain and reduce inflammation, and they aren't expensive. But if your joints are chronically sore—a side effect of pushing hard—you may find yourself taking these medications almost daily. That puts you at risk for a range of problems from stomach upset to intestinal bleeding. Ideally, you want not only to block pain and stop the condition from getting worse, which are the common goals of pharmaceuticals, but also to encourage body processes that make your condition better.

Certain natural therapies can safely block pain and reduce inflammation, as well as support the repair of injured soft tissues and help prevent further damage to them. Europeans have used them for years; Americans

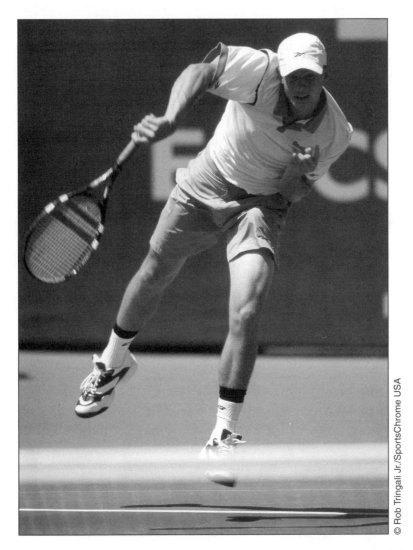

© Rob Tringali Jr./SportsChrome USA

Look for patterns in your diet that may dispose you to mineral deficiences.

are late adopters, hesitant to stray from familiar painkillers. As an athlete, you need to get beyond that fear of the unknown to maintain a high level of conditioning well past middle age (whenever that is). A little science may help.

Natural therapies appear to work for a number of reasons:

• They inhibit the enzyme cyclooxygenase-2 (COX-2). COX-2 facilitates prostaglandin production; prostaglandins contribute to pain and inflammation. Aspirin and the other NSAIDs do the same thing.

• They suppress tumor necrosis factor (TNF-a) and interleukin-1B. Keeping the level of TNF-a down in an injured or arthritic joint allows joint damage to heal. Similarly, the less interleukin-1B that's produced in your body, the less inflammatory response your body will have to tissue damage.

• They suppress leukotriene B4, which attracts inflammatory cells, such as white blood cells, to a damaged area.

• They promote the synthesis of glycosaminoglycans (GAGs) in the joints. These chemical chains—"glyco," as in *glycogen*, and "amino," as in *amino acid*—play an important role in the functioning of cartilage. The GAGs bind to protein cores to form proteoglycans, and these molecules suck up water like a sponge, which gives the cartilage its squishy texture and its ability to cushion your bones.

• They suppress the cartilage-destroying enzymes collagenase, which degrades collagen, and phospholipase. Collagen is a fundamental part of skin, tendons, blood vessels, and bones; you obviously don't want collagenase around them. Phospholipase breaks down other components of connective tissue.

• They attract water to the cartilage to enhance synovial lubrication. Joints are bathed in synovial fluid; water is a major component of the fluid.

In terms of blocking action, then, a natural therapy aims to inhibit cyclooxygenase so that you don't form prostaglandin, a source of pain and inflammation; to suppress TNF-a and interleukin-1B, which also pump up the inflammatory response; and to suppress cartilage-destroying enzymes. On the positive side, the goal is to promote synthesis of glycosaminoglycans and proteoglycans, because they are important in forming cartilage and keeping it spongy so that it can absorb shock.

The chart in table 3.3 provides an overview of supplements for the joints. Consider the long-term value of these products, and choose one or an affordable combination of complementary substances. If you want to have as much fun moving your body later as you do now, you need to protect your cartilage, ligaments, tendons, and bursa.

Table 3.3 The Joint Supplement Chart

Supplement	Function(s)	Dosage	Cost	Comments/ cautions
Boswellic acid	Acts as an anti-inflammatory; suppresses *leukotriene* synthesis	500 mg/day	90 tablets (250 mg): $16 Monthly cost: $5	
Bromelain	Reduces swelling and inflammation; accelerates tissue repair	300–500 mg/ day based on 2,000 GDU/ gram (Bromelain's potency is measured in gelatin-digesting units, GDU)	60 tablets (500 mg): $12 Monthly cost: $6	Bromelain is often thought of only as a digestive aid. It is a collection of protein-digesting enzymes found in pineapple juice and stems. It might amplify the effect of antibiotics, so don't combine the two.
Cetylmyristoleate (CMO)	Improves joint articulation and reduces inflammation	300 mg/day (based on a study in which osteoarthritis sufferers took two 75-mg capsules A.M. and P.M.)	180 capsules (60 mg): $100 Monthly cost (study dosage): $100 Some dosage recommendations are 1–3 gm/day, so the cost can be higher.	The study on CMO conducted by the San Diego Clinic showed notable results. The two non-responding subjects had suffered previous liver damage from steroid use or alcohol abuse.
Chondroitin sulfate	Slows joint deterioration by interfering with enzymes that help the breakdown process; reduces pain	400–1,000 mg/day	60 capsules (400 mg): $14	In Europe, chondroitin sulfate is widely used in a form that can be injected into joints; in the U.S., that option is rarely available.

(continued)

Table 3.3 *(continued)*

Supplement	Function(s)	Dosage	Cost	Comments/ cautions
Copper	Strengthens connective tissues	2–4 mg/day	Monthly cost: $14 100 tablets (2 mg): $6	Take copper between breakfast and lunch with chromium.
Fish oil and flaxseed oil	Suppresses the production of inflammatory mediators such as *prostaglandins* and *leukotrienes*	2 tbs./day, or 2 capsules/ day	Monthly cost: $3.50 100 capsules (1,000 mg): $10	
Gamma-linolenic acid (GLA)	Reduces swelling and tenderness in joints by suppressing an inflammatory response	400–600 mg/ day	Monthly cost: $6 60 capsules (300 mg): $20	GLA is a fatty acid found in evening primrose oil, borage oil, and black currant seed oil. It has been used to suppress chronic inflammation.
Glucosamine	Serves as a primary building block of the substances that make up cartilage and *synovial* fluid; specifically, your body uses it to make *glycosaminoglycans*	1,500–3,000 mg/day	Monthly cost: $20 90 capsules (1,000 mg): $36	Your body produces glucosamine, but adding it to your diet is an effective way to boost your body's ability to keep your cartilage spongy. About 90% of what you take in is actually absorbed.
Methylsulfonyl-methane (MSM; aka methyl sulfone or dimethylsulfone, DMSO2)	According to patents, serves in multiple ways: reduces arthritis pain and inflammation and supports tissue regeneration	100–1,000 mg/day, depending on the severity of symptoms; usual dosage is 500 mg/ day	Monthly cost: $54 250 capsules (500 mg): $15	Research with MSM is weak; the claims of patent holders are primarily bolstered by anecdotal evidence.

Supplement	Function(s)	Dosage	Cost	Comments/cautions
Oligomeric proanthocyanidins (OPCs)	As antioxidants ("free-radical scavengers"), boost the body's immune response to inflammation	150–300 mg/day	Monthly cost: $2 60 capsules (100 mg): $45	OPCs are flavonoids found in many plants and in red wine; supplements contain extracts from grape seeds or pine bark. Used in Europe for decades. Pycnogenols is the name given by the developer, a researcher at the University of Bordeaux in France, and trademarked by Horphag Overseas Limited of Geneva. Don't take aspirin with it; the two together can cause excessive bleeding.
S-adenosyl-methionine (SAMe)	Appears to reverse damage caused by *TNF*, blocks enzymes that degrade cartilage, and protects *proteoglycans* to keep cartilage spongy	600–1,200 mg/day to start for 2 wk., then 400 mg/day (study dosage)	Monthly cost: $45 60 tablets (200 mg): $50 Monthly cost (after 2-wk. start period): $50	Many of the potent claims about SAMe come from a study published in the *British Journal of Rheumatology* in 1997.

This overview is just a hint of what you can use in an effort to reinforce your joint and bone health. Many product formulas combine several of the therapies and include vitamin C, an important antioxidant, but review what each one is supposed to do for you before you invest in such a product. At the very least, pay attention to your minerals, described earlier in this chapter, and bolster the aid to your joints with glucosamine and chondroitin sulfate if you can afford them.

Jim Warren, who has trained such superstars as home run hitter Barry Bonds and is also the founder of a supplement company called Team Pro2, notes that the higher daily amounts of glucosamine and chondroitin would apply to world-class/high-mileage athletes who have symptoms of joint damage. Even at the elite level, however, athletes who feel 100 percent would take the lower dosage. By explaining how to use his product, Jim sheds light on the factors you need to consider in finding a product that matches your needs with your bank account and then deciding how much of the product to use:

> Our suggested daily serving for Glucosamine Sport Plus is 1,000 milligrams (four tablets at 250 milligrams each). We are able to achieve the same results with a lower amount because of the other synergistic ingredients, such as digestive enzymes (creating easier delivery of very stable and hard-to-absorb glucosamine and chondroitin) and herbs. The herbs we use have ibuprofen-like qualities (anti-inflammatory and pain relief) and also address other issues that can cause pain, such as lack of circulation. As the category evolves, more companies are starting to add the [same] ingredients. Most companies stuck with glucosamine and chondroitin only to hold down cost, but ultimately a formula such as Team Pro2's ends up costing less because you use less product.
>
> In some instances, such as my own situation—aged 44 with significant structural damage—athletes may need to use six tablets a day (three twice a day) for the 1,500 milligram total amount. Dosage tends to be personal. Most people feel a change in three to five days.

A League of Its Own: Glutamine

Glutamine is categorized as a nonessential amino acid, because the body can synthesize it. That classification is misleading, however. Every cell in your body uses glutamine, and maintaining an ample supply—which is crucial for supporting your immune and cardiovascular systems, building muscles, replenishing glycogen levels after exercise, protecting your brain from ammonia toxicity, and much more—can take special dietary efforts. If you don't have enough of it, your muscles will begin to atrophy, and you may even get sick. Take a look around you at the athletes who succumb to infections after a marathon or while training heavily for a big game. Strenuous exercise can lead to rapid glutamine depletion. After a hard day in the gym or on the field, your glutamine stores could drop by 40 percent or more, opening the door to overtraining syndrome.

Your body so desperately needs glutamine that when supplies do plummet it will extract other amino acids from your muscles and try to manufacture the lost molecules. Your body plunges into a catabolic state. Do this to your body repeatedly, and you will put yourself in an over-trained state for weeks at a time.

Both plant and animal proteins contain glutamine, so protein recovery products of all kinds provide this amino acid. If you opt for a carbohydrate recovery product, as many endurance athletes do, look for glutamine as well as the BCAAs. As an example, Team Pro2 Pro Recovery & Strength powder includes a gram each of glutamine and the BCAAs in one scoop, even though the powder is very low in protein.

The final issue, of course, is how much to take. Most of the glutamine you ingest goes straight into the lining of your intestines to act as intestinal fuel and to produce certain substances that the body requires. Glutamine increases the number of lymphocytes and macrophages (immune cells). Knowing this, companies may include what appear to be high dosages in their products; alternatively, you may see a substance called lysophosphatidyl choline (LPC) used (Stryer 1995). LPC increases the intestinal wall's ability to pass nutrients, such as amino acids, to the bloodstream.

You may want to take glutamine both before and after workouts, but taking it afterward is what you need most. The amount usually recommended is two to three grams daily, after a workout, but as you'll see in the next chapter, "Supplementing for Strength," athletes of 300 pounds sometimes boost the dosage to five grams (Rohde, Maclean, and Pedersen 1998; Castell, Poortmans, and Newsholme 1996).

As a hard-working athlete trying to make performance gains, focus your thinking and financial resources on recovery products before anything else. If you don't counter the glycogen depletion, muscle breakdown, fluid loss, and mineral imbalances caused by intense training, your hard work will only tear your body down. You could end up a physical wreck, more susceptible to sickness and injury than many of your weekend warrior friends. Watch your performance soar and feel immediate benefits when you invest wisely in recovery products as a complement to a balanced diet.

CHAPTER 4

Supplementing for Strength

Your strength depends on your muscles, bones, joints, and energy. This chapter looks at strength-building supplements and at diets specially designed for strength athletes, so that you can figure out exactly what you need to achieve your muscle development goals and become more powerful.

It also covers supplements that can help you stay powerful. Athletes training for strength commonly have a high rate of injury, from muscle and cartilage damage to concussions. While the nature of the training program certainly plays a role both in staying injury free and in building functional strength, specially formulated food products can also help you do both.

Muscle-Building Supplements— In the Eyes of the NCAA

In a summer 2000 revision of its bylaws, the National Collegiate Athletic Association (NCAA) implied that nutritional supplements, such as those described in this chapter, provide muscle-building and muscle-sustaining benefits to athletes. The NCAA researched available evidence and decided the following:

> The NCAA Division I board of directors . . . agreed that muscle-building supplements are performance-enhancing and provide a competitive advantage to those institutions that can afford to provide these supplements to their student-athletes (NCAA 2000).

This rationale stands behind the NCAA's directive that Division I schools may not provide muscle-building supplements to athletes. A close look at the supplements labeled "nonpermissible" by the NCAA provides good background for understanding the sample diets for elite strength athletes that are presented later in this chapter.

Amino Acids

This category comprises two notable parts of a strength athlete's diet: glutamine, given its rightful prominence in the discussion of recovery products; and branched chain amino acids (BCAAs) (Garlick and Grant 1988). Glutamine is included on the nonpermissible list largely because some athletes use it in a loading program similar to a creatine loading program. Just before a competition, they take relatively large amounts combined with high-glycemic carbohydrates to get a pump. This is not the suggested use, which is post-workout.

Your body makes glutamine, but you can add to your supply with plant and animal protein, which also provide BCAAs. Found in dairy products and red meat more than in other whole-food protein sources, BCAAs insure against muscle breakdown and preserve muscle glycogen stores (Bloomstrand, Hassmen, and Ekblom 1991). So, if you're in a Division I school, drink your milk.

Chrysin

This supplement was patented in Europe in the mid-1990s after some studies pointed to its value in minimizing the conversion of testosterone to estrogen, a natural process called aromatization. For this reason, it is sometimes used in conjunction with a prohormone, such as Androstenedione, to get the maximum benefits of the testosterone-boosting supplement. If the dosages attributed to some European elite athletes is correct—one to three grams of chrysin a day—then this supplement is very expensive. It is typically sold in quantities of 60 tablets of 250 milligrams each for $25, which translates to $100 per month for two grams per day. Add that to the $50 per month or more that you spend on the complementary Androstenedione products and the 25 milligram per day dosages of DHEA (dehydroepiandrosterone)—both of which are hormone precursors of testosterone—and the investment in testosterone boosting becomes substantial.

Chondroitin and Glucosamine

Chondroitin sulfate slows joint deterioration and reduces the joint pain associated with injury and cartilage degeneration. American athletes should heed the more extensive experience that Europeans have with chondroitin and accept it as a valuable natural joint therapy. This same comment applies to glucosamine, which helps keep cartilage spongy and also made the NCAA's nonpermissible list.

Creatine

Creatine phosphate occurs naturally in the body. Its main function is to replenish energy in the muscles. When you have a quick-energy need, your anaerobic system breaks down creatine phosphate to resupply ATP to your muscles. This system delivers a great boost if you have an intense short-term need, but the ATP supplied from it is depleted after eight to ten seconds of all-out activity. Creatine products are designed to boost the body's reserve of usable creatine phosphate for energy. As a corollary, they can contribute to an increase in muscle size—a creatine pump—and can improve muscle performance. Creatine does not affect testosterone levels. (See the sidebar "Creatine Loading: Feeding the Body's Quick-Energy System" on page 22.)

Creatine products have become much more sophisticated and useful to athletes over the years. FSI Nutrition, for example, has attempted to increase the absorption rate of creatine with its effervescent creatine, which has a patented delivery system. FSI's description of the value of its creatine product to strength athletes clarifies one reason why the NCAA sees it as a muscle-building supplement:

> The performance benefit of effervescent creatine is the increased ability to do high-intensity, short-term work. This is the same benefit seen with creatine monohydrate, just to a significantly greater degree. The stimulus of increased training leads to a true muscle hypertrophy, not just water swelling or "volumization." The improvement in AWC [anaerobic work capacity] shown in the pilot study performed at Creighton University by Dr. Jeff Stout was 195 percent over a creatine monohydrate and 84 percent over a creatine monohydrate/carbohydrate blend (Sakurada, Pharm, and Carnazzo 1999).

Athletes who use creatine may gain important related benefits, particularly in helping to protect the brain after a head injury (Sullivan et al. 2000). The mechanism of protection follows the same course in the muscles as it does in the brain. When you work out, oxygen is depleted from the muscle, which then burns the creatine. Similarly, in a head trauma, oxygen is depleted in the brain. The brain must burn something; if you have a relatively high level of creatine in the brain, it will burn the creatine before it burns tissue.

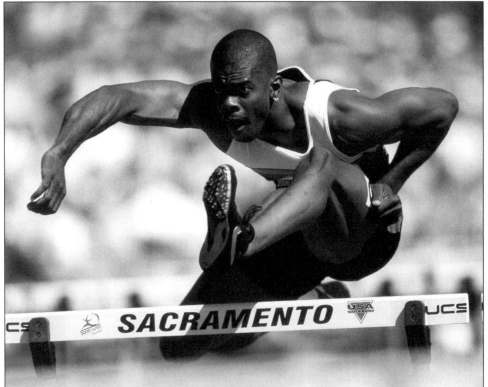

The Sporting Image/Tony Duffy

The NCAA tries to ensure "fair play" by holding down the number and type of supplements that schools may supply athletes.

Ginseng

In terms of muscle-building action, there is speculation that ginseng helps restore muscle glycogen and high-energy phosphate compounds to normal levels, but no research to date really supports that hypothesis. It's usually discussed seriously in the context of stimulants rather than muscle-building products.

Glycerol

Glycerol is a liquid that is used in medicines and cosmetics. Sometimes, you will also see it as the liquid in a creatine monohydrate suspension. Also known as glycerin, glycerine, and glycerate, you will see it as the mystery ingredient in many protein bars (see the protein bar chart in table 4.1). Glycerol is generally assigned the same four calories per gram as carbohydrates, but because it has characteristics of lipids (fats) and carbohydrates, that number may change. It makes bars a little moister and provides energy without causing blood sugar to spike. It's used as a

Table 4.1 The Protein Bar Chart:
A Comparison of Content and Best Uses

Product (company)	Total calories	Protein (gm)	Protein sources (in order of listing)	Carbs (gm)	Fat (gm)	Best uses/ comments
Big 100 Food Bar (MET-Rx)	320	27	Milk protein isolates, caseinate, whey protein concentrate, egg white, and glutamine	48	2.5	Meal replacement
BioProtein (MLO)	300	21	Whey protein concentrate, milk protein isolate, soy protein isolate, hydrolyzed protein, and egg albumin	39	7	Meal replacement
Bio-X (Absolute Nutrition)	320	27	Whey protein concentrate, milk protein isolate, and egg albumin	41	4.5	Meal replacement
Designer Whey (Next Proteins)	260	30	Whey protein concentrate, hydrolyzed whey protein, and whey protein isolate	6	4.5	Post-workout snack; 75 cal. from *glycerine*— not a carb, but in metabolic terms, an equivalent
Extra Protein (Sportpharma)	290	31	Milk protein isolate, hydrolyzed protein, whey protein isolate, and caseinate	11	6	Post-workout snack; 70 cal. from *glycerine* (see pg. 74)
GeniSoy (GeniSoy)	220	14	Soy protein isolate	34	3.5	Meal replacement; not all flavors okay for vegans

(continued)

Table 4.1 *(continued)*

Product (company)	Total calories	Protein (gm)	Protein sources (in order of listing)	Carbs (gm)	Fat (gm)	Best uses/ comments
KetoPRO (MET-Rx)	250	34	Milk protein isolates, caseinate, whey protein concentrate, egg white, glutamine, and hydrolyzed protein	13	8	Meal replacement or snack for a *ketagenic* dieter (lowers carbs and ups consumed fat to reduce body fat.)
Lean Body (Labrada)	300	30	Whey protein concentrate, whey protein isolate, hydrolyzed whey protein, milk protein isolate, and caseinate	19	7	Meal replacement; balance of calories from alcohol, depending on flavor of bar
Meso-Tech (MuscleTech)	340	25	Whey peptides, whey protein concentrate, whey protein, soy protein isolate, and caseinate	44	7	Meal replacement
Muscle Recovery (Pharmavite)	180	15	Whey protein isolate, caseinate, soy protein isolate, hydrolyzed protein, and milk protein isolate	12	4.5	Post-workout snack; 30 cal. from *glycerine* (see pg. 74)
Myoplex HP (EAS)	250	20	Whey protein isolate, milk protein isolate, caseinate, and soy protein isolate	30	5	Post-workout snack; contains creatine

Product (company)	Total calories	Protein (gm)	Protein sources (in order of listing)	Carbs (gm)	Fat (gm)	Best uses/ comments
Myoplex Lite (EAS)	190	15	Milk protein isolate, whey protein isolate, caseinate, and soy protein isolate	27	3.5	Post-workout snack; Lite refers to percent of calories and fat in relation to Myoplex Deluxe
Myoplex Deluxe (EAS)	340	24	Whey protein isolate, caseinate, and milk protein isolate	44	7	Meal replacement
Premier Eight (Premier Nutrition)	270	31	Caseinate, whey protein isolate, soy protein isolate, and whey protein concentrate	8	6	Post-workout snack; 60 cal. from *glycerine* (see pg. 74)
Pro Blend (Human Development Technologies)	290	30	Caseinate and hydrolyzed protein	16	5	Meal replacement; 60 cal. from *glycerine* (see pg. 74)
Promax Bar (Sportpharma)	280	20	Whey protein concentrates and caseinate	36	5	Meal replacement
Protein Fuel (Twinlab)	320	35	Soy protein isolate, whey protein isolate, whey protein concentrate, caseinate, and hydrolyzed protein	12	5	Meal replacement or post-workout snack; 80 cal. from *glycerine* (see pg. 74)
Protein Plus (MET-Rx)	300	32	Milk protein isolates, caseinate, whey protein concentrate, egg white, glutamine, hydrolyzed protein, and whey protein isolate	15	8	Meal replacement or snack for a *ketagenic* dieter (see pg. 74)

(continued)

Table 4.1 *(continued)*

Product (company)	Total calories	Protein (gm)	Protein sources (in order of listing)	Carbs (gm)	Fat (gm)	Best uses/ comments
Protein Plus (PowerBar)	290	24	Whey protein isolate, caseinate, and soy protein isolate	38	5	Meal replacement
Protein Revolution (Low Glycemic Technologies/ MET-Rx)	230	22	Hydrolyzed protein, caseinate, soy protein isolate, and whey protein isolate	2.5	8	Meal replacement or snack for a *ketagenic* dieter (see pg. 76); 60 cal. from *glycerine* (see pg. 74)
Pure Protein (Worldwide Sport Nutrition/ MET-Rx)	290	34	Caseinate, hydrolyzed protein, and whey protein isolate	15	5	Meal replacement
Steel Bar (American Body Building)	315	16	Milk protein isolate, whey protein concentrate, and caseinate	50	5	Meal replacement; most carbohydrates from sugars
Ultimate Lo Carb (Biochem/ Country Life)	230	20	Soy protein isolate and whey protein concentrate	2	6	Meal replacement or snack for a *ketagenic* dieter (see pg. 76); 60 cal. from *glycerine* (see pg. 74)
Ultimate Protein Bar (Biochem)	290	30	Whey protein isolate, caseinate, and hydrolyzed protein	19	4.5	Meal replacement; 50 cal. from *glycerine* (see pg. 74)

Notes: (1) New terms are italicized and defined. (2) If use is "meal replacement," you could use half as a post-workout snack. (3) Trademarked terms and other names or phrases with more marketing value than substance have been omitted. (4) These bars are not recommended as preworkout energy bars. (5) Many of the bars contain sugar. Others use aspartame or stevia as sweeteners.

component of sports drinks because it causes cells to hold water; therefore, it may help delay dehydration during exercise and promote rehydration afterward. The bodybuilding community has generated a buzz about the substance having unique value in pumping up before a contest, but the evidence is anecdotal. The bad buzz is that glycerol can cause severe headaches, nausea, diarrhea, and vomiting.

HMB

HMB refers to beta-hydroxy beta-methylbutyrate monohydrate, which is a byproduct of the body's normal breakdown of leucine, one of the branched chain amino acids. As with creatine, supplementation is used to boost the body's own supply to enhance performance. In this case, supplementation supports the body's ability to minimize muscle breakdown, build muscle, and decrease body fat. HMB supplements are intended for use with a high-protein diet supporting very strenuous exercise.

L-Carnitine

Although L-carnitine is often labeled an amino acid, technically speaking it is not one. It is actually more like a vitamin, and your body makes it out of lysine and methionine, which are amino acids. L-carnitine helps transport fatty acids across the inner membrane of the mitochondria, subcellular structures that body cells need to metabolize food into energy sources. Athletes generally use L-carnitine to support fat burning and efficient energy production, not muscle building, although research doesn't support that it aids fat loss, either.

Melatonin

A hormone produced naturally in the body, melatonin helps regulate sleep/wake cycles. In the late 1990s, it gained a lot of popularity as a cure for jet lag, inducing a natural sleep on demand. Because your muscles grow when you're resting, melatonin could have a peripheral connection to muscle building. It also has a reputation for provoking vivid, pleasant dreams, which may be a side benefit that some athletes value over more muscle mass. On the other hand, too much melatonin can potentially cause adverse reactions such as lethargy and disorientation. Just because a substance is classified as a dietary supplement doesn't mean you can't overdose on it; follow the guidelines on dosage on the label.

POS-2

POS-2 is a product made by Advocare rather than a supplement. It is part of a series called the Performance Optimizer System. The ingredient list of POS-2 includes creatine and amino acids, which is why it made the nonpermissible list.

Protein Powders

This category encompasses the many prepackaged recovery products, customized blends of selected proteins and flavorings, and meal replacement powders in which more than 30 percent of the calories come from protein. The value of these products to muscle building, and the debates concerning their relative values, are covered in detail in chapter 3.

Tribulus

Tribulus terrestris is an herb that some European studies have linked with elevation of testosterone levels. The manufacturers' recommended dosage of 500 milligrams per day is also supposed to keep testosterone levels up on a continuing basis once they're elevated, so some people use it to enhance sexual performance. Don't expect that outcome, however, because research doesn't support it.

Supplements That Stayed off the List

The NCAA did make exceptions for certain supplements containing proteins if they met all of the following conditions:

• The supplement must fall into one of the following categories: vitamins and minerals; energy bars; calorie replacement drinks, such as Ensure and Boost; or electrolyte replacement drinks, such as Gatorade and PowerAde.

• It must not contain additional ingredients that are designed to assist in the muscle-building process, such as any of the substances listed in the nonpermissible list.

• No more than 30 percent of the calories may come from protein (based solely on the package label). By this standard, any of the bars on the energy bar chart in chapter 2 would be acceptable, but most of the protein bars on the chart in table 4.1 would not. The exceptions are some of the meal replacement bars: Bio Protein, GeniSoy, MesoTech, Myoplex Deluxe, Steel Bar, and ProMax Bar.

Beyond Nonpermissible: The Banned Boosters

In addition to the list of supplements that Division I schools may not provide to athletes, some muscle-building substances are completely banned from college athletics. The list of agents is long and includes illegal substances such as anabolic steroids, but it also includes currently legal substances called prohormones, which are discussed in chapter 6. Androstenediol, Androstenedione, Norandrostenediol, and DHEA (dehydroepiandrosterone) fit into this category, and many products contain or feature them, including those that package a couple of them together in a "testosterone stack." On a positive note, these products appear to be safer than anabolic steroids as long as they are not overused. On a discouraging note, you may get some of the same cosmetic side effects that afflict anabolic steroid users, such as bad skin, hair where you don't want it, and hair loss where you do want something to comb. These results are one reason why athletes like to combine prohormones with chrysin, which reportedly mutes some of these side effects by minimizing the conversion of testosterone to estrogen.

A Personal Reflection on Steroid Use

I want to add a personal note about anabolic steroids, because I was a bodybuilder in the nutritional Dark Ages—the days before high-quality, specially formulated food products and supplements were accessible. It was hugely frustrating to me to enter a show with my trainer and gym pals saying I was destined for a win, only to be edged out by someone using steroids. I'd close my eyes backstage and know that my nemesis was the gal with the deepest voice.

Throughout this competitive period in the mid-1980s, I was surrounded by the attractive performance benefits of anabolic steroid use. For one thing, overtraining was no longer a concern; men and women around me lifted heavily day after day. Feeling strong consistently and doing well in contests helped them ignore pesky side effects, such as dramatic changes in their genitals, uncontrolled mood swings, high blood pressure, and nasty acne. Why didn't I join them in realizing the short-term benefits of steroid use—in getting a few more trophies and bigger applause? First, it seemed like more fun doing it the hard way, and second, I was writing about bodybuilding as well as enjoying it. Through research and conversations with insiders, I grew to realize that the day was coming when the legal and healthy options for strength athletes would be extraordinary. The time has arrived. Paired with an excellent diet, the off-the-shelf products available today are putting natural bodybuilders on top and supporting amazing gains by clean athletes in all strength sports.

Competitive Strongmen and Strongwomen: The Training Diet

America's Strongest Man in 1999, Bryan Neese, has a relatively simple nutritional program to achieve his strength goals. His diet, which is covered in detail in chapter 2, emphasizes beef and the Pro Blend products he uses as protein sources. He takes three supplements to protect and build his muscles—glutamine, branched chain amino acids, and creatine; his quick energy source is products with herbal stimulants and Androstenedione; and he rounds out his eating with lots of vegetables and complex carbohydrates.

Bryan may joke that his beef eating reflects the dietary habits of his home state of Indiana—"the strongest state in the nation"—but as a sports food, beef is no joke. With a biological value of 80 (which means that a relatively high proportion of the protein is retained in the body), beef has a great ability to fuel muscles with the nitrogen they need for development. And lean cuts of beef have a high concentration of B vitamins, iron, zinc, and phosphorus:

- B-1 (thiamin) helps convert carbohydrates to energy.
- B-2 (riboflavin) and B-3 (niacin) also help convert the food you eat to energy.
- B-6 (pyridoxine) helps synthesize amino acids and break them down into useful compounds.
- B-12 (cobalamin) is an important player in DNA metabolism, red blood cell formation, and the health of your central nervous system. (By the way, there are no plant sources of B-12, but some fermented foods such as miso and soy sauce have some B-12. *If you're a vegetarian strength athlete, be sure to take a B-12 supplement.*)
- Iron is critical for energy production and other metabolic functions.
- Zinc is key in breaking down and utilizing carbohydrates and in synthesizing protein.
- Phosphorus is important for strong bones and teeth as well as for energy metabolism.

Beef can also inhibit your performance if you eat it at the wrong time. It sits in the gut a lot longer than fish, for example, or the protein sources in sports supplements, so it is not part of an ideal pre-competition meal. During your event, you don't want your body energetically trying to digest a steak when it's supposed to be sacking a quarterback. Also, watch your portions, even if the beef is lean. I think that Barry Sears' guidance on animal protein is a good one: At a single meal, the portion should not be larger than the palm of your hand. And, yes, if you have a big hand, you get a bigger portion than your teammate with the average-sized hand. For health and performance reasons, you would be better off dividing that monstrous hunk of meat and eating it at meals that are a few hours apart rather than devouring it all at once.

You'll see many similarities between Bryan's diet and that of Linda Holland, who became the national champion at the North American Strongman Society (NASS) Strongwoman Nationals in 2000—even in terms of calories. Six feet tall with a competitive weight of only 145 pounds, Linda must be converting food to raw power, because it certainly isn't converting to the saddlebags that plague many other 46-year-old women.

Her accomplishments in the Strongwoman Nationals included pulling a 4,800-pound truck 40 feet in 17 seconds and an event called the "carry and drag"—carrying 165 pounds of weight between her legs for a distance of 40 feet and then, for the return trip, grabbing the handles of a metal sled loaded with 460 pounds and dragging it backward to the starting line. She did that in 72.9 seconds.

In some ways, the basic diet that supported her training, as well as her decade of power-lifting training and competition, is unique to her personal tastes, especially her consumption of milk—nearly a gallon a day. It isn't fat-free milk either. Linda drinks whole milk and eats about six to eight whole eggs a day. That's about 150 grams of fat (1350 calories).

In other ways, Linda's whole-food diet seems like the ideal strongman diet designed by Chad Coy: It consists of lots of protein and fresh vegetables, six to seven meals a day, and heavy supplementation with glutamine and creatine. Chad is research and development director for Human Development Technologies and is ranked among the top strongmen. His ideal diet follows these guidelines:

- Your daily food intake should be split into five to seven meals.

- Protein should make up 30 to 40 percent of the total calories. Concentrate on low-fat protein: Drop the heavier meats such as sausage, bacon, and hamburger (unless it is 92-percent lean). Don't even eat lean beef a couple days before a show or competition, because it takes too long to digest.

- Carbohydrates should make up 40 to 50 percent of the total calories. Carbohydrates are the body's preferred fuel source. Strength athletes commonly run out of gas quickly, because they think that protein is the prime and only macronutrient they need. Focus on starch, fiber, and fruit. Eat a number of different carb sources such as whole grain breads, pasta, rice, oatmeal, yams, and any fruits and vegetables.

- Fats should make up 10 to 20 percent of the total calories. Although you want to limit fat intake, you need a certain amount to maintain health and strength. For example, fat donates the backbone for all steroid hormones, supports joint health and brain function, and moves the fat-soluble vitamins (A, D, E, and K) through your body. It's best to eat lean and consciously add good fat such as flaxseed oil or an EFA (essential fatty acid) supplement to your diet.

• Water is the most overlooked nutrient. Both protein and fat metabolism depend on water; without adequate water, carbs cannot be stored properly. Drink half your bodyweight in ounces of water: If you weigh 200 pounds, drink 100 ounces (three liters) of water daily, or about 12 glasses. You need more if you drink beverages with caffeine or take creatine. You need less if you eat a lot of water-rich foods such as fresh fruits and vegetables, or if you drink fresh juices.

Chad feels strongly that most of your focus should be on whole food, but sports foods and supplements have valuable functions in your strength-building diet. He says,

> I would like to eat all of my food, but that would be impossible for me! I am forced to use supplements in order to get the number of meals in a day that I need. The ones I use make up for food. I use Pro Blend-55, Pro Blend Bar, MRP-44 [all three are from Human Development Technologies], and from time to time a carb supplement like Carbo Force [American Body Building] or CarboPlex [Unipro].

Chad also uses supplements to support specific goals he has as a strength athlete. A sample strength-building daily diet that includes these supplements for an athlete of 250 pounds or more is found on page 86.

This sample diet raises a number of key points about supplementing for strength:

• You can overuse creatine. Even for a 250-pound athlete, 10 grams of creatine can be a large amount and may result in problems, such as cramping and bloating, unless you're adequately hydrated. Linda Holland, who weighs about 100 pounds less than Chad, takes the same amount of creatine monohydrate twice a day with no ostensible problems. Keep two things in mind, however. First, chronic, excessive use of creatine monohydrate can affect the receptor sites you need to absorb it. You will find yourself needing to take more to get the same effect. One approach is to use it during the competitive season and drop it from your menu during the off season. Another is to use a relatively low maintenance dosage after a one-week period of loading, as described in chapter 1. Second, if you take more than you can use, you may not suffer side effects, but you will excrete the extra. Consider using a delivery system like effervescent creatine that should make dosages above five milligrams unnecessary.

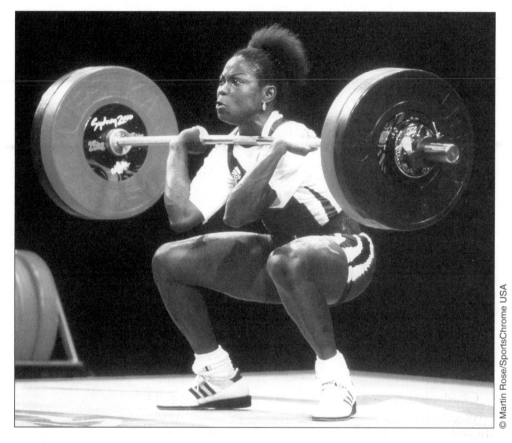

© Martin Rose/SportsChrome USA

Muscles, joints, the anaerobic energy system—strength athletes eat to keep all of them pushing hard.

• The amount of glutamine you need can vary. Both Chad and Linda take glutamine twice a day—early in the day and after their workouts. They each take five grams per serving, which is much more than the normally recommended two-gram dosage for most athletes in training. The appropriate amount corresponds to individual needs, which are influenced by stress levels, disease, and other conditions. Hospitalized patients have been aided by glutamine dosages of 20 to 40 grams. Unless you are training hard for a big event like a power-lifting or strongman competition, the recommended amount plus a protein-rich diet should give you what you need. Again, as in the case of creatine, don't waste your money by giving your body more than it can use.

• The right fat will help you build up. Flaxseed oil gained more recognition in the late 1990s, after many athletes began to realize that not all fats are enemies of athletic excellence. Flaxseed oil contains linoleic acid and alpha lineolenic acid (ALA), both of which are essential fatty acids with great value to strength athletes. They suppress the production

Sample Strength-Building Daily Diet for a 250-Pound Strongman

	Calories	Protein (gm)	Carb (gm)	Fat (gm)
Meal #1 (about 7:00 A.M.)				
12 egg whites	204	42	4	
3 servings oatmeal	435	16	77	7
Piece of fruit (e.g., apple)	84	21		
24 oz. water, along with				
10 gm creatine				
1 multivitamin				
5 gm glutamine				
1 tbs. flaxseed oil	117			13
Meal #2 (midmorning)				
Meal replacement shake	297	44	26	2
Protein meal replacement bar	280	32	16	5
Water				
Meal #3 (lunch)				
2 grilled chicken breasts	770	116	30	
2 c. (cooked) rice	640	12	140	
1 c. vegetables (e.g., broccoli)	44	4	7	
Water and supplements same as Meal #1	117			13
Meal #4 (midafternoon, before training)				
Meal replacement shake	297	44	26	2
Piece of fruit	84		21	
Water and supplements:				
5 gm ribose				
5 gm glutamine				
3 gm BCAA				
a thermogenic aid (not more than the recommended amount)				
Meal #5 (late afternoon, after training)				
16 oz. grape juice and supplements:	300	2	74	
5 gm ribose				
5 gm glutamine				
10 gm creatine				
4 scoops of whey protein powder	360	70	8	6

Meal #6 (dinner)

2 c. (cooked) pasta	420	12	88	2
1 large salad	111	3	9	7
12 oz. turkey	500	102		10

Totals (numbers are rounded)

Calories	5,000
Protein	40% of calories; 2 gm per pound of body weight
Carbohydrates	45% of calories
Fat	15% of calories

Data courtesy of Chad Coy, M.D. Labs, Tempe, Arizona.

of substances that contribute to inflammation in damaged joints. They also synthesize hormones, reduce cholesterol, and support strong immune responses. If you want to integrate flaxseed oil into your diet without gulping down a tablespoon or taking a few capsules, you can use it as a salad dressing. Small amounts of the valuable ALA also show up in soy, canola, and walnut oils.

• Ribose can be a good extra. Ribose is a sugar that forms the base of ATP, and it's usually taken right before a workout and within 30 minutes after a workout to aid recovery. The usual manufacturers' recommended amount is about half of Chad's five-gram dosage, since he designed his diet for a very large man—himself.

• You need a healthy way to add calories. Both Chad and Linda rely on meal replacement powders to add quality calories for two meals a day. Linda mixes hers with milk to boost her total calories.

• Too much fat will get in your way. Chad's thermogenic aid—basically, an aid to fat burning—is Thermic Blast Capsules (from Human Development Technologies). He takes the recommended amount of two capsules for explosive energy. The composition and use of such products and their role in boosting lean mass and dropping unwanted weight are explored in detail in chapter 6, "Gaining or Cutting Weight."

• HMB is a finishing touch. Although Chad does not include it in his strongman diet, Linda takes three grams of HMB (four capsules three times a day) to reduce the muscle breakdown caused by her heavy workouts. HMB receives more attention in the football player's daily diet described in the following section.

The NFL Pro's Preseason Diet

Professional athletes in high-dollar, high-visibility sports such as football and basketball have various coaches and nutrition gurus who design training and eating programs specifically for them. Athletes may deviate from their programs occasionally—a couple beers, a Philly cheese steak—but the pros know that their routine of eating and supplementation can boost their value to the team. They have compelling financial and performance reasons to stick with it.

For a high-end view of how performance-enhancing products can fit into a daily diet, consider the following preseason program. EAS, a leading sports supplement company designed it for one of the NFL's rising stars. The player used it successfully prior to the 2000 season.

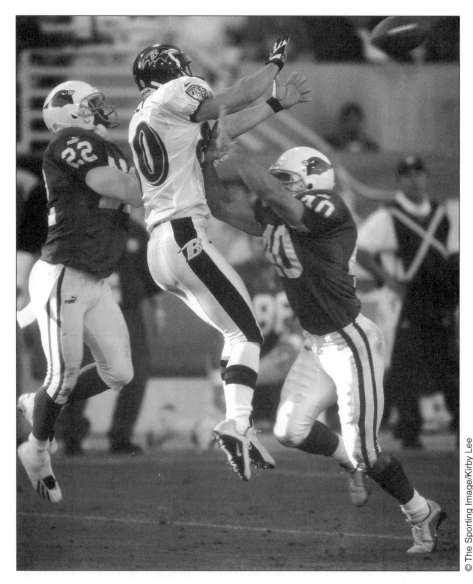

© The Sporting Image/Kirby Lee

The investments involved in a professional football career warrant dietary discipline and supplementation.

Performance-Boosting Diet for a Pro Football Player

Meal #1 (breakfast)

1 cup cooked oatmeal

6 to 8 egg whites or Egg Beaters

16 ounces water

1 capsule AAB (Athlete's Antioxidant Blend)

Antioxidants help neutralize the free radicals that result from intense exercise.

2 capsules Structured EFA

Essential fatty acids support a strong metabolic response to intense exercise, helping the body produce hormones, repair muscle tissue, metabolize insulin, and burn fat.

2 capsules Multi-Blend

A good multivitamin/multimineral formula supports metabolic functions for athletes at all levels.

2 capsules Glucosamine HCL

An integral part of all connective tissue in the body, glucosamine helps prevent and even repair breakdown associated with high-impact activities; research shows that it is more effective as an anti-inflammatory substance than ibuprofen.

Meal #2 (midmorning snack)

1 serving packet Myoplex Deluxe in water

This meal replacement is designed to support athletic performance; essentially, it's a healthy convenience. Rather than a meal replacement, which is the product classification, you might actually think of it as an extra meal. Much like the strongmen and strongwoman described previously, a professional football player needs a couple thousand high-quality calories more than most people to build and maintain muscle and to keep energy high.

4 capsules HMB

Meal #3 (lunch)

two 6-ounce chicken breasts

1 cup steamed vegetables

1 cup steamed rice

16 ounces water

same supplements as in Meal #1

Meal #4 (afternoon snack)

Note: Depending on your training schedule, you may choose to switch this meal with Meal #5, the post-workout snack. Regardless of the order, the meals should be separated by at least a couple of hours.

1 serving packet Myoplex Deluxe in water

4 capsules HMB

Meal #5 (post-workout snack)

1 serving packet Myoplex Deluxe in water

1 packet Riboforce HP in water

This patented creatine-ribose formula is designed to take advantage of a synergistic relationship between creatine and ribose, which are both important to energy production.

Meal #6 (dinner)

8-ounce filet of chicken or fish

1 baked potato or 1 cup steamed rice or pasta

salad or steamed vegetables

16 ounces water or, for a change, a diet soda or equivalent

same supplements as in Meals #1 and #3

Meal #7 (bedtime snack)

1 scoop of Precision Protein in water

A high-quality protein repairs and builds muscles for hard-training athletes. Don't expect to see performance benefits, however, unless you are putting a great deal of effort into your training.

4 capsules HMB

2 scoops CytoVol in water

Designed to produce an optimal cellular environment for new muscle growth, this important amino-acid formula supports your immune system.

5 capsules ZMA HP

Strenuous exercise often causes deficiencies in zinc and magnesium and these losses compromise muscle growth and function and negatively affect the immune system. Quality of sleep is a big issue associated with the deficiencies; it often can be immediately remedied with the appropriate dosage of these compounds.

The football player's preseason diet follows the same distribution of macronutrients as the strongman's year-round training diet, but the calorie total is slightly lower:

Calories	3500
Protein	40 to 45 percent of calories, or 1.5 grams per pound of bodyweight
Carbohydrates	40 to 45 percent of calories
Fat	10 to 15 percent of calories

Courtesy of Rob Fulcomer, EAS, Inc, Golden, Colorado.

Every strength athlete can learn from a model program like this one. It demonstrates balance for a strength athlete, yet it includes ample protein to meet the higher requirements related to strenuous training and competition. The following sections provide some key insights about the supplements used in the model program.

Dosages

The dosages used in the model program don't necessarily match the recommended amounts on the bottle. With the exception of glucosamine, they are actually less than the manufacturer's recommended amounts, because the three Myoplex Deluxe shakes per day meet some of the needs that the other supplements address. The glucosamine dosage is somewhat higher than the standard recommendation, because the athlete is a very large, professional football player who requires the additional amount.

Brands

If you seek the full range of benefits from performance-enhancing products—energy and recovery, as well as general health—then you need to know the synergistic and antagonist relationships among components and formulas. If you have put yourself on the track to becoming an elite athlete, then you must face this challenge. In the beginning, unless you have a background in nutrition or physiology, working out an entire program of food and supplements is often easier if you rely on a single point of contact, such as a customer advisor at a company with a comprehensive product line. EAS supports a 24-hour hotline staffed by people with generic and brand-specific product information. A one-brand regimen may not ultimately be the ideal program for you, but it will give you the foundation for understanding how to make adjustments. In the meantime, you probably won't spend as much money on products that duplicate benefits or counteract each other.

Cost

You probably want to know what this NFL pro would pay for the products on his daily list. The following breakdown is based on the retail cost of products in 2001 found on the **netrition.com** website:

Product	Per month cost
AAB	$40
EFA	$45
Multi-Blend	$40
Glucosamine HCL	$50
Myoplex Deluxe	$240

HMB	$60
RiboForce HP	$75
Precision Protein	$75
CytoVol	$30
ZMA HP	$25
Total monthly cost:	$680

Customizing to Fit Your Budget

If this program represents the ultimate, what should someone aspiring to be an elite or professional athlete incorporate to improve? In other words, what should you back out first if you have financial constraints? Logically, the initial way to address the financial concern is to point out that a diligent strength athlete of any level would be eating about six meals a day, so in most cases the cost of a meal replacement is actually less than the cost of a whole-food, high-protein meal. If you spend about eight dollars per day on meal replacements, consider what you would spend on whole food (including the investment of your time in preparation) and ask yourself if the cost is really outside your budget.

If you factor in those issues and still find that you need to cut costs, then the product that you should probably back out is HMB. It is expensive, and it is a refinement in a nutritional program. In addition, you need use it regularly to feel the value of it; if you slack off periodically because of cost, you undercut your investment. If your budget continues to choke you, you may have to leave the RiboForce behind until you are closer to competition time, when it can give you a competitive edge.

If you are launching a new program and committing yourself to more demanding workouts, be careful about removing other components from the program. When you suddenly begin to train hard, your immune system can be compromised. The regular workouts will ultimately strengthen your immune system, but with noble goals and insufficient planning, you might push too hard in the first few weeks. As a result, the high-intensity training will break your body down. You'll get sick and not show up in the gym for a couple of weeks. By the time you return, you'll be frustrated and want to embark on an aggressive program to make up for lost time. You can predict the outcome: a repeat of the previous cycle. Some of the elements of the sample diet program boost your immune system while you get acclimated to a tougher workout. CytoVol, for example, is intended to keep the immune system strong during strenuous workouts. None of these supplements are a substitute for good planning, however: Ease into greater intensities. Take the stairs one at a time.

As you plan your training menus to include supplements and other sports foods, take your current body size into consideration. You may want to end up a 250-pound strongman, but don't ask yourself to eat like one if you're only 180 pounds. Get yourself in the best shape possible through training and eating at your current weight, and then move upward by incrementally adding more—more weight in the gym and more calories in your meals. Even if you have the financial resources to afford everything the pros use, you should still start with the basics and then add a product at a time, so that you develop a keen sense of how the different supplements affect your body. Your log and food chart will help you keep track of the effects.

Finally, good timing is vital to success. Follow the manufacturer's directions on when to take each product to get maximum benefits.

CHAPTER 5

Adding Endurance

This chapter is about using sports foods to support your endurance training, not to substitute for it. If you can't complete a one-hour run without sucking down energy gel, you aren't ready for a marathon. Your endurance program needs to train your body to use stored energy sources. You then supplement those sources when your body has difficulty keeping up.

The average person stores between 1,500 and 2,000 calories, enough fuel for a 20-mile run—if you're a well-trained athlete who has adapted to using energy reserves efficiently. If you hit the wall at the 20-mile mark, your body is reacting normally to a depletion of your muscle glycogen stores. At that point, even elite athletes might turn to a product containing simple sugars to keep them going. If you hit the wall at mile 10 in a marathon, however, you're trying to do too much too soon.

After years of diligent training, you may have learned that your body can go long distances on city streets, dirt hills, or kilometers of ocean, but you may still not know what foods your unique body needs to make the going easier. Following in the footsteps of many elite athletes, you must begin a process of trial and error to find out which foods and supplements keep your energy steady without causing gastric distress and which ones undermine your performance.

Begin your search for that ideal formula with liquids. Unless you tackle ultramarathons, adventure races, or other endurance activities that last more than a day—activities that are covered primarily in chapter 7—you may be best served by liquid nutrition.

To push through exercise that lasts a few hours, endurance athletes generally need to ingest carbohydrate drinks or other products that provide a minimum of 45 grams of carbs (180 calories) per hour after the first hour of activity. Athletes whose events commonly last longer than a day tend to add protein to diets that carry them through long training sessions and events. During training and competition, endurance athletes need about .75 grams of protein per pound of bodyweight per day—

1.2 to 1.4 g/kg of bodyweight—to maintain a positive nitrogen balance and to promote muscle recovery and growth.

Regardless of whether you go with a product that contains all carbs or with one that offers a balance of carbs, protein, and fat, you'll need to ascertain the product's digestibility, ability to sustain energy, and total calories. The basics of these issues are covered in chapter 2.

Carbohydrate Drinks: The Basic Difference

When you choose a drink or decide how much to dilute a premixed liquid supplement to make it suitable for your use, you should know the logic underlying the design of sports drinks. (These criteria hold true for powders that you mix yourself, too.) First, a quality sports drink stimu-

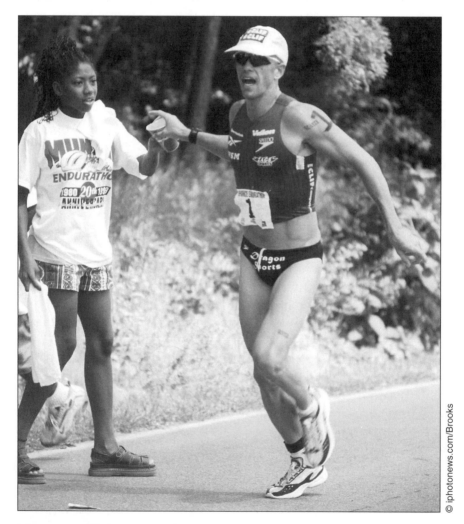

© iphotonews.com/Brooks

Liquids are an efficient way of pumping carbohydrates and electrolytes into your body when you're on the run.

lates rapid fluid absorption; your body absorbs it more quickly than plain water. Second, it helps you hold on to the fluid, because it provides sodium and helps you avoid depleting your glycogen stores. Use the following guidelines on carbohydrate concentration to evaluate these drinks in terms of absorption:

• Before and during exercise, choose a drink with a low carbohydrate concentration (about 4 to 7 percent). At higher concentrations, you may have a hard time digesting the carbohydrates and water quickly enough to use them immediately, and the drink may undermine your performance. You can calculate the concentration by dividing the weight of the carbohydrate in grams by the weight of the liquid in grams. For example, if an eight-ounce serving of a sports drink gives you 14 grams of carbohydrates, you need to turn the ounces into grams—a weight measure—by multiplying 8 (ounces) by 31.1 (the number of grams in one ounce):

$$8 \times 31.1 = \textbf{248.8 grams}$$
(the weight in grams of an eight-ounce serving), and

14 grams is the weight of
the carbohydrates in the eight-ounce serving, so that

$$14 \div 248.8 = .056, \text{ or } \textbf{5.6 percent carbohydrate concentration.}$$

• Choose drinks with a higher carbohydrate concentration for carbohydrate loading or for use after you exercise.

Table 5.1 offers some insights into the differences between premixed carbohydrate drinks.

Fixing Your Own Drink

One elite ultra-runner and multisport adventure racer, Lisa Smith, backs up an astonishing list of endurance accomplishments with a masters degree in health education and fitness, so she is a rich source of advice on eating for endurance. She offers the following general guidance for someone who is preparing to do an endurance event:

> I think most people going into races these days tend to overeat in the days and weeks before an event. They think, "I have to load up! I have to eat so much to store what I need." If you eat a normal diet, your body already has many stored nutrients. In preparing for a race, just be normal. Don't try to eat four times as much the day before. Like those pasta parties—I raced horribly after something like that.

Table 5.1 Premixed Carbohydrate Drinks

Premixed drink (company)	Calories (per 8 oz. unless noted)	Carbo. profile	Carbo. concentration (per 8 oz.)	Electrolytes	Comments
AllSport (Pepsi)	70	High fructose corn syrup	8–9%	55 mg sodium 55 mg potassium	Carbonated
Endura (Health World Limited)	62	Glucose polymer-fructose	6%	90 mg sodium 180 mg potassium	• Registered in Australia as a therapeutic sports drink • Also contains magnesium, the absorption of which is decreased by sodium
Extran Liquid Energy Food Boxes (Nutricia/ Royal Numico)	320 per 6.75-oz. box	Glucose syrup (a proprietary mix of long-chain complex carbohy- drates)	[Not a valid point of comparison for this product, which is primarily complex carbohy- drates]	20 mg sodium	• Primarily for elite endur- ance athletes; popular among Tour de France cyclists • Recom- mended amount is 1 box/hr. during intense events • In U.S., has FDA designa- tion as a food • Only 6% simple sugars by weight
Gatorade (Quaker Oats)	50	Sucrose, glucose, and fructose	6%	110 mg sodium 25 mg potassium	Through sponsorship of events—large and small—it is often the drink available along the racecourse; if so, try it before the event to know how your body responds

Premixed drink (company)	Calories (per 8 oz. unless noted)	Carbo. profile	Carbo. concen- tration (per 8 oz.)	Electrolytes	Comments
PowerAde (Coca-Cola)	70	High fructose corn syrup and malto- dextrin	8%	55 mg sodium 30 mg potassium	

At this point in her competitive career, Lisa no longer eats any type of energy bar or gel in competition, although she sometimes grabs an energy bar for a snack during light training times. Her reason is twofold: After years of eating energy bars, she got sick of them, and she found that liquid nutritional supplements work better for her during serious training and competition. Her preferred supplementation for training and competition is a mix of a meal replacement powder and a carbohydrate-electrolyte drink. Together they deliver 300 calories in a half-liter sport bottle. Lisa says, "I've done an entire 50-mile race only on these drinks and not eaten anything."

Combinations like this one seem to be gaining popularity among cyclists, long-distance runners, duathletes, and triathletes. Steve Fluet, a five-time All-American triathlete, has coached a number of champion endurance athletes, and he says that combining a protein drink with a carbohydrate drink works very well for athletes "who find themselves getting a little hypoglycemic with the carb drink alone." Some of the athletes he coached felt lightheaded when they tried to rely solely on carbohydrate products during two- to three-hour training sessions, so Steve added protein and a little fat to their drinks to slow down the absorption of sugars, and the combination worked well.

To duplicate the kind of mix Lisa and Steve achieve, you could take one product from column A in table 5.2 and one from column B, but be careful to match the total amount of powder you use with an appropriate amount of water. For example, if you mix Metabolol and Cytomax, keep in the mind that the usual mixes are two scoops of Metabolol in 12 ounces of water and one scoop of Cytomax in 16 ounces (roughly one-half liter) of water. Experiment with the mix, adjusting the concentration so it isn't too strong or too weak.

Some experts would go beyond pedestrian terms like "strong" and "weak" and point to potential problems with *osmolality* (particles/kilogram of water) or *osmolarity* (particles/liter of solution) with this kind of mixing. These two measures, both of which gauge particle concentrations

Table 5.2   Ad Hoc Product Combinations for Endurance
Athletes

Column A	Column B
Meal replacement powders with these characteristics: • Low fat • 50–55% of calories from carbs • 30–40% of calories from protein • Targeted to serious endurance athletes	Carbohydrate drink powders with these characteristics: • A mix of complex carbohydrates (most likely maltodextrin, which gets glucose into the bloodstream without causing an energy spike) and sugars • Low protein (carbohydrate-to-protein ratio around 4:1) or no protein • Low or no fat • Electrolyte replacement • Targeted to serious endurance athletes
Cytomax Pre-Formance (Cytosport) Metabolol Endurance (Champion Nutrition)	10-K (Kenwood Spring Water/Suntori) Cytomax (Cytosport) 85% carbohydrates Endurox R⁴ (Pacific Health Labs) 75% carbohydrates (you might also want to mix this with a higher carb product) Extran (Royal Numic/Nutricia; sole U.S. distributor is Zoeller Marketing) 100% carbohydrates Extreme Fuel (Symmetry) 100% carbohydrates contains herbs Prolyte Energy Drink (Prolyte) 100% carbohydrates contains caffeine Pro-Endurance (Team Pro2) 88% carbohydrates Revenge (Champion Nutrition) 80% carbohydrates contains caffeine (you might also want to mix this with a higher carb product) Zing (Zing, Inc.) 100% carbohydrates

in diluted solutions, are essentially synonymous concepts. Marketing literature may use these terms to emphasize the science behind the product. The osmolality or osmolarity of a product can help you set expectations, but in terms of your own performance, the manufacturer's by-the-book numbers may or may not have practical relevance. You have to try the product to see how you respond during your particular activity.

If a manufacturer does follow defined osmolarity levels, you can expect to have no cramping or other digestion-relation distress for several hours. Osmolarity strongly influenced Nutricia's design of Extran, a popular competition drink among top European cyclists. Extran's formula is 80 percent complex carbohydrates and only 20 percent simple sugars. Once Nutricia's blend is dissolved, the osmolarity of the product is relatively low. This low particle concentration enables the manufacturer to dissolve a relatively large quantity of carbs per milliliter of water before there is any danger of the product causing intestinal cramping.

On the other hand, if a product has by-the-book osmolality values, after that initial period of high performance you may experience a downturn. The big variables again are the product itself and how you use it. You may not absorb fluids as well after several hours; you need something in your gut to open up the blood vessels a bit. Clearly, you want maximum blood flow to your muscles during exercise, but without a little going to your gut as you take in nutrients, you will experience some cramping.

Refer to table 5.2 for types of meal-replacement and carbohydrate-drink products that might be combined. Note that these products are not the only ones you can combine if you feel a little lightheaded, or hypoglycemic, when you ingest carbohydrate drinks.

Innovation in Premixed Drinks

The serious product-development research in this category of sports supplements is successfully addressing osmolality, ways to avert cramps, and many other issues that endurance athletes have long tried to handle through trial and error. A prime example is the effort that Michael Zumpano, founder of Champion Nutrition, has invested in creating a drink that attempts to help average athletes strengthen their metabolic weak links so that they can perform more like genetically gifted endurance athletes. As Michael explains,

> I was headed toward medicine, but I didn't like being around sick people all the time. One summer, I worked with a doctor and cried myself to sleep every night. Little children falling out of trees, or getting gangrene and losing an arm. One beautiful 17-year-old

girl—her brothers talked her into going logging and a log rolled over her foot. She lost her leg up to the knee. Horrible things everyday. I said, "I can't live like this. I want to devote myself to improving the situation for healthy people."

Michael turned to athletes, people who naturally excelled and had physiological gifts, and studied them. He focused on people who developed faster and recovered better than other people. He felt that the simple explanation of their performance—superior genetics—was not an answer that would help other athletes improve. Equipped with a physics and mathematics background, he dove right into the science and concluded that genetics expresses itself through metabolism. After asking himself, "What is it that's different about the metabolism of elite athletes?" he came up with the notion of metabolic optimization:

Metabolic optimization is the concept of looking at how these genetically elite athletes work and trying to mimic that in a normal person. So we are optimizing a normal person's metabolism to look like the metabolism of someone who's genetically superior.

That's only half the picture that Michael saw, however. The other half was creating food products that would enable an athlete to consume calories as efficiently as possible. At first, Michael was just trying to feed himself something that would make him visible enough to get a date: A sophomore in college and 6'3", he weighed a measly 121 pounds. He was taking between 18 and 24 credit hours each quarter in core subjects, and he felt he didn't have time to stop and eat, so he attempted to concoct things that would sustain him.

The year was 1977, and one of the aspects of nutrition that began to interest Michael was how to increase the amount of creatine phosphate in muscle. He found that an ingredient called succinate seemed, if taken before an activity, to affect performance positively, resulting in more energy, more oxygen, and no soreness after a brutal workout. Michael didn't necessarily know all the science at the time, but his empirical evidence was later backed up by studies (Brooks and Fahey 1984). Those studies confirmed that succinate could be provided in a formula that increased muscles' use of glycogen and creatine phosphate, two important energy substrates. It also improved oxygen uptake, so that the athletes felt like they got more wind, and it helped avert soreness by mitigating the tearing effect of calcium ions on muscle tissue.

Consequently, even before Michael officially founded Champion Nutrition in 1986, he had elite endurance athletes using this first succinate product, called Muscle Nitro. Two decades after he began his research, many endurance athletes at the top of the rankings turned to a new

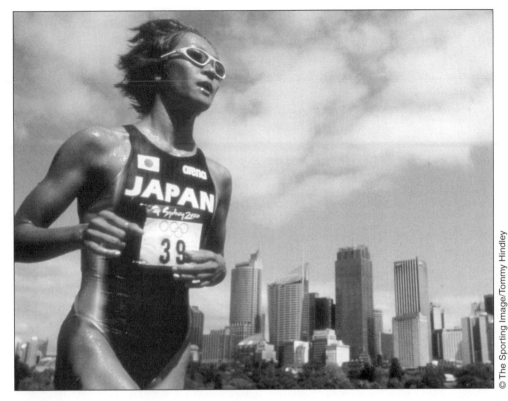

Endurance athletes need high-quality protein after a workout to prevent muscle breakdown.

Champion product, a drink called Revenge, which was designed to improve oxygen delivery during an event. The thinking behind it is intriguing. Here's a small piece of it in Michael's words:

> We thought of the deformability of red blood cells. People with sickle cell anemia, for example, don't have deformable red blood cells—they can't mash down and squeeze through capillaries as well [as a normal person's], and when they do, they don't have as much contact with the surface of the capillaries, so that they don't exchange as much oxygen and CO_2.

Michael suggests that taking Revenge for a minimum of four days in a row will improve the deformability of red blood cells. The result would be getting more oxygen released from the blood cells and more carbon dioxide (CO_2) exchanged, although the proof at this point is primarily anecdotal.

The formula also aims to reduce the formation of lactic acid so that there is no need to buffer it after it's made; the objective is to keep energy substrates in the muscle. Another objective goes back to the design of

Muscle Nitro: Champion attempted to discover how to give endurance athletes that second wind right from the start.

For any athlete, that elusive second wind is the pacing you get a few minutes or a few miles into a race. Your systems feel as though they are finally running smoothly and synergistically. At the start of the activity, that pacing is blocked by adrenaline—even if you aren't nervous. When you first start an activity, even if you just go from walking to jogging, your body puts out adrenaline. The adrenaline causes the blood vessels to clamp down and restrict the flow of oxygen. All of a sudden, when the adrenaline subsides, your blood vessels relax and you get a better supply of oxygen.

When he created Revenge, Michael consciously sought a formula that would prevent adrenaline from causing the blood vessels to clamp down. His intention was to give athletes their second wind immediately. Just as Brian and Jennifer (Biddulph) Maxwell had to go through multiple PowerBar formulas, however, before they arrived at something the normal human stomach could not only tolerate but also appreciate, Michael also had to go through several formulas for Revenge so that athletes' taste buds wouldn't reject the project outright. As he puts it,

> We have to coat the ingredients because they taste so bad. We pushed the limits of flavor technology in developing this product. We tried to develop a new technology in order to make a coating fine enough so that it wasn't gritty. We ran out of money when the machine was half finished.

The machine was later created to refine the taste of Revenge, but Michael went ahead and introduced it with its gritty texture and found that athletes adopted it despite the drawbacks. Interestingly enough, they were doing precisely what Lisa Smith and Steve Fluet described—taking the product and mixing it with another liquid to produce the kind of drink that satisfied their energy needs, was absorbed easily, and seemed to produce results they needed in the long haul. And they made it taste good, or at least, good enough.

Averting Endurance Problems

With endurance athletes, the concern ranges from too much to not enough. Too much water and not enough sodium results in hyponeutremia. Too much carb concentration in a drink produces cramps. Not enough electrolytes triggers fatigue, tremors, diarrhea, and nausea. Too much food before an event causes sluggishness and stomach distress. Not enough calories before an event makes an athlete bonk. To get the full benefit of information in this chapter, combine it with the insights throughout the book on the full range of energy and recovery needs for endurance athletes. Here's an overview of key points:

- In the hours before an intense endurance event that will last less than a day, any food you eat must be highly digestible. Avoid red meat, which takes a long time to digest, and fatty foods like cheese. You also don't want these foods the day before an event.

- If good fats such as flaxseed oil are part of your regular diet, continue to ingest them as you would normally.

- Eat to keep your blood sugar regulated; high-glycemic foods will sharply affect your insulin levels.

- Do not do creatine loading, because the loading causes your muscle tissue to retain excess fluid, creating a creatine pump. Small amounts of creatine in energy and recovery products will benefit your performance, however.

- Use carbohydrate gels to restore glycogen levels during training or competition that exceeds 90 minutes. For some athletes this can drop to an hour.

- Take in amino acids after endurance training or an event to prevent muscle breakdown; focus on glutamine and the BCAAs.

- Water alone isn't enough to support your full recovery after an intense endurance workout or competition. Use an electrolyte-replacement product to help restore your mineral balance.

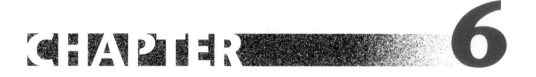

CHAPTER 6

Gaining or Cutting Weight

For an athlete, gaining weight means adding lean muscle mass, and most of the time cutting weight means dropping fat. The only time weight loss involves a deliberate effort to reduce muscle mass is when an athlete tries to shift from bodybuilding or a strength/mass sport like football to an endurance sport like long-distance running. With this premise as a foundation, this chapter examines the products designed to help you shift your body composition by adding lean muscle, cutting fat, or doing both.

The Mantra of Many: "Get Bigger"

Eating protein does not increase muscle size in adults, nor does it even keep muscles the same size. Resistance exercise, using your own bodyweight or external weights, stimulates muscles to grow or to maintain their size, and that development is supported metabolically by eating protein. Other nutrients have specific roles in that growth, too.

In trying to put on lean mass, you have to have some patience, even if you are using high-quality supplements. If you're under 25, you may be able to stimulate growth at the rate of about one pound every 8 to 10 weeks without doing anything except working out and eating well. As you get older, that growth rate becomes harder to achieve; in fact, you may take twice as long to achieve the same one-pound gain if you're in your 30s. Protein products, amino-acid supplements that feature glutamine and branched chain amino acids, and minerals should support faster gains if (and only if) you combine them with a base diet that supports your goal.

To calculate how many daily calories you need to gain lean mass, multiply your current weight by 20 and then add 1,000 calories. For example,

$$170 \text{ pounds} \times 20 = 3,400 \text{ calories;}$$

$$3,400 \text{ calories} + 1,000 \text{ calories} = 4,400 \text{ calories.}$$

The source of these calories is very important. Even though your aim is adding muscle, you don't want the entire caloric increase to come from protein. One approach to gaining lean mass relies on maintaining a relatively high carbohydrate intake—65 percent of calories—with protein at 15 percent and fat at 20 percent. Some sport scientists have found that keeping carbs high while eating one gram of protein for every pound of bodyweight supports lean mass gains in many athletes. If you have never tried putting on mass before, you may want to try this program, particularly if you play a sport that requires a weight gain while it demands lots of energy. Some bodybuilders also adhere to these ratios.

The following example shows the 65-15-20 approach for a 170-pound athlete who wants to add lean mass:

Total daily intake during weight-gain phase:	4,540 calories
Total carbohydrates:	737 grams (4,540 calories × .65 = 2,951 carb calories. Each gram of carbs yields four calories, so that's 2,951 carb calories ÷ 4 = the number of carb grams needed, or 738 grams)
Total protein:	170 grams (one gram per pound of bodyweight)
Total fat:	101 grams (101 × 9 = 909 fat calories)

In contrast, many bodybuilders and strength athletes take an approach that is higher in calories and protein. During the gain phase, these athletes might add 2,000 to 2,500 calories to their daily intake, with some of the increase coming from carbohydrates, such as rice, pasta, and potatoes, to help keep their energy high for intense workouts. They would also consume two or more grams of protein per pound of bodyweight. With this program, protein sources deliver about one-third of the daily calories, carbohydrates contribute 50 to 55 percent, and fat accounts for 15 to 20 percent.

The following example shows the 55-30-15 approach for a 170-pound athlete who wants to add lean mass:

Total daily intake during weight-gain phase:	4,540 calories
Total carbohydrates:	624 grams
Total protein:	340 grams (two grams per pound of bodyweight)
Total fat:	76 grams

This high-calorie, high-protein regimen has supported tremendous gains for Mohamad (Moe) Moussawi, who began his bodybuilding career as a middleweight and moved up to capture heavyweight titles. Moe left Lebanon for the United States after winning that country's top amateur bodybuilding title at the age of 18. During that same year, 1992, he clinched the middleweight title at the Lebanese wrestling championships and took second place in the middleweight division of the Lebanese

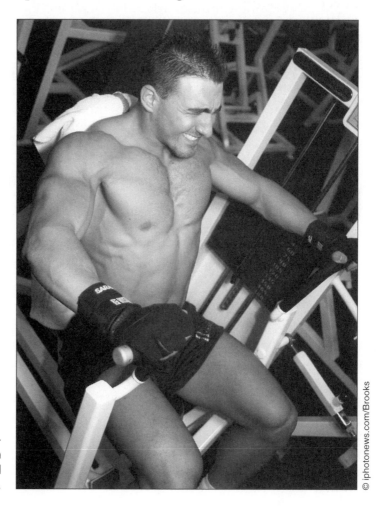

Gain muscle by harmonizing protein consumption and resistance exercise.

© iphotonews.com/Brooks

power-lifting championships. After laying off for three years while he got on his feet financially in the United States, Moe resumed his drive to win bodybuilding awards through a completely natural program. In 1997, he took home trophies as the overall novice and middleweight champion at the Musclemania show. In 2000, he captured the Mr. California overall title as a heavyweight. Table 6.1 shows how the statistics changed over time for this 5'10" athlete.

In this same period, a predictable gain for a natural athlete without the scrupulous use of performance-enhancing supplements would have been about 10 to 18 pounds. To some extent, Moe's incredible jump to a prime, heavyweight physique reflects a genetic predisposition to muscle building, but more than that, it highlights his disciplined and intelligent use of whole foods and sports foods.

As owner of a supplements store, Moe's Muscles, Moe has access to nearly everything on the market. He has personally tried many of the products he sells, and he notes that he had several short-lived experiences with supplements:

> I'm sensitive to a point that when I take a different supplement, I can tell if it's better or if it's less effective than another one. Because I keep it natural, my body can tell me what's going on. If you use a lot of steroids, your system is messed up.

Moe is so careful about what he ingests that, before accepting sponsorship from a supplement manufacturer, he has sent products to a lab for independent testing. Staying natural means that quality is essential to the kinds of gains that make him competitive.

Like every bodybuilder on the rise, Moe follows an off-season diet that builds size and pre-competition diets that help him melt fat and make him ripped. Each contains a different distribution of macronutrients and

Table 6.1   Competition Comparison

1997 Musclemania	2000 Mr. California
Weight: 201 lb.	Weight: 235 lb.
Body fat: 6%	Body fat: 5%
Biceps: 19"	Biceps: 20"
Waist: 29"	Waist: 28"
Chest: 51"	Chest: 52"
Quads: 28"	Quads: 28"
Calves: 17"	Calves: 17"

supplements, with the mass-building program much heavier on supplements than the on-season program. On the off-season diet, Moe uses creatine, a weight gainer, and joint supplements in addition to Androstenedione, Androstenediol, Norandrostenedione, nor-Androstenediol, or a similar testosterone booster. (These prohormones are discussed later in this chapter.) Like many other natural bodybuilders, he has tried just about everything on the shelf to try to achieve the size results that anabolic steroids engender. He says,

> I even used DHEA at one time, and it did boost my testosterone level a little bit, but honestly I did not feel good with it. It's more for people who are a little bit older than I am. The manufacturers do say it's good for people who are over 40 years old.

On an average day during the off-season, here is how Moe's nutritional program supports gains:

Sample Off-Season Daily Menu to Gain Lean Mass

Meal #1 (about 7:00 A.M.)

large egg-white omelet

mashed potatoes

Meal #2 (about 9:00 A.M.)

Next Proteins Designer Protein shake (40 grams of protein)

As an alternative, Moe sometimes adds a carbohydrate to the shake (for example, a banana) or uses a weight gainer by Next Nutrition, Big Whey. (See table 6.2 in this chapter for more information on weight-gain products.) At some point in the morning and afternoon, Moe adds a joint supplement, such as glucosamine/chondroitin sulfate, and doses of pro-hormones—specifically, Androstenedione and Norandrostenedione.

Meal #3 (about 11:30 A.M.)

16 ounces of chicken breast

lettuce with lemon

You may substitute a white fish like orange roughy or halibut for the chicken.

Meal #4 (about 1:30 P.M.)

pasta or rice

Moe often keeps protein and complex carbohydrates separate during the off-season. This food-combining strategy reflects the theory, advanced in the mid-1900s by Dr. William Hay, that mixing the two may lead to inefficient digestion and gastric

(continued)

(continued)

problems because the body digests proteins differently from complex carbohydrates, or starches. You may want to test this formula personally before rendering judgment.

Meal #5 (about 3:30 P.M.)

Designer Protein shake (40 grams of protein)

10 grams creatine

Moe has used different creatine products, primarily MuscleTech's 6000ES with amino acids and Extreme Sports Nutrition's Extreme Creatine Monohydrate. He firmly believes that creatine has value for a bodybuilder only during the off season, because of the water retention it causes. This seasonal use of creatine does not necessarily apply to strength athletes such as football players and athletes in other contact sports, however.

About one and one-half hours later, at roughly 5:00 P.M., Moe does weight training for one and one-half hours.

Meal #6 (immediately following the workout; about 6:30 P.M.)

Designer Protein shake (up to 65 grams of protein)

10 grams glutamine

10 grams BCAAs

10 grams creatine

Moe notes that his post-workout protein shake contains more protein than the two he ingests earlier. He sums up the debate about how much is too much in this logical way: "Some people believe that your system does not absorb more than 35 or 40 grams at one time. I'm one of the people who believes it depends on how much you work yourself and how much your body needs at that specific time."

Meal #7 (between 8:30 and 9:00 P.M.)

1 can of tuna (or other protein snack, such as turkey, salmon, or other fish)

Meal #8 (bedtime)

4 capsules Z-Mass PM (Cytodyne)

Courtesy of Moe Moussawi, founder of Moe's Muscles.

Moe is a big fan of this combination of zinc aspartate and magnesium aspartate, referred to as ZMA by other manufacturers. BALCO Labs licensed its ZMA formula to several manufacturers, including Cytodyne and EAS, so that the products from these companies are fundamentally alike, although packaging and recommended dosages may vary a bit. Bodybuilders like Moe use it "to get growth hormone levels higher."

This function has been substantiated in research conducted by Dr. Lorrie Brilla, a sports performance researcher at Western Washington University. After monitoring a group of competitive NCAA football players who took ZMA nightly for eight weeks during spring training, she found that they showed two and one-half times greater muscle strength gains than the players taking placebos. She concluded that the strength increases were linked to anabolic hormone increases. The free and total testosterone levels of the players taking ZMA rose significantly—by 30 percent—as compared to the 10 percent *decreases* in the placebo group during the eight-week spring-training/test period. Insulin-like growth factor-1 (IGF-1) also rose in the ZMA group, but dropped 20 percent in the players taking the placebo. Moe also highly recommends the sleep benefits of ZMA. It brings on a restful, dream-filled sleep that many athletes describe as very pleasant.

Moe's daily intake is 5,000 to 6,000 calories on this diet. Protein from egg whites, chicken, fish, and protein shakes provide around 35 percent of the calories. Later in this chapter, you'll see that his program to get ripped for a contest involves meals that contain fewer total calories, a higher percentage of protein, fewer carbohydrates, and less fat.

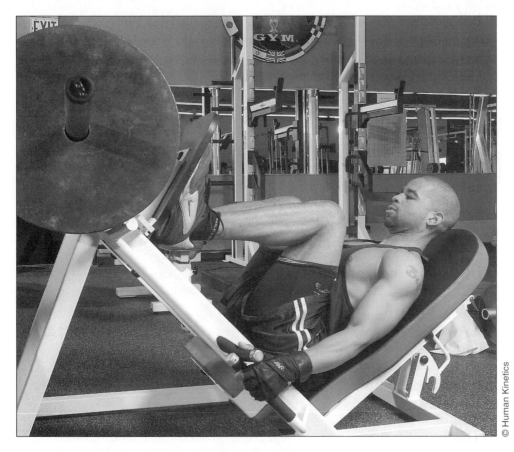

© Human Kinetics

Use weight gainers carefully so as to realize the results as muscle instead of fat.

Regardless of your stage of development, take a cue from Moe's use of weight gainers. Moe works in the product once a day at most, a program that precisely reflects what many top manufacturers recommend. Even if you're skinny with ambitions of gaining size as quickly as possible, overuse of weight gainers or a bad choice of product will add excess fat to your body in addition to the muscle mass you're building.

To avoid bad choices, keep a close eye on serving sizes and ingredients. Servings of weight gainers are typically measured in scoops, and the scoops in many tubs hold around 30 grams of product. You can't squeeze a lot more calories into that scoop unless you add fat. You can add more calories to a two- or three-scoop serving, however, if you increase the size of the scoop. With some weight gainers promising more than 2,000 calories in a single three-scoop serving, you may open the tub and find a soup ladle. In addition, some so-called weight gainers are the powder equivalent of ice cream smothered in chocolate sauce. Your goal is lean mass, so too much fat and simple sugar will not help you make the kind of gains you desire.

Table 6.2 will help you evaluate the formulas in selected weight-gain products. Be sure that your extra calories come from sports foods that meet the following criteria:

• Your body can easily absorb them. Look for a product with high-quality protein and low saturated-fat content.

• They deliver calories in quantities that your body can handle efficiently. Don't force-feed yourself. Your body can only comfortably handle around 600 calories at one time, and when you overdo that—think of a huge holiday meal—you may be headed for an upset stomach as well as poor nutrient uptake. Big meals also slow your metabolism, causing you to store more of the calories as body fat. If you really like the formula and taste of a product that advertises an extremely high calorie count per serving, try using a half serving for a couple of weeks, and then check your gain. One to two pounds would be a good gain. If you didn't achieve that amount, then bump up your serving size to the recommended level.

• They rely more on low-glycemic carbohydrates than on simple sugars. When you see glucose or sucrose prominently mentioned in the list of ingredients, you are looking at a product loaded with simple sugars. They will trigger an insulin surge, which could send you through an energy high and then a low, encouraging your body to store excess sugar as fat.

You may prefer to make your own weight-gainer product by starting with high quality protein or protein products and then adding low- to moderate-glycemic carbohydrates and essential fatty acids. If you use a

Table 6.2 The Weight Gainers Chart

Product (company)	Calories per serving (in water unless noted)	Serving size (gm)	Macronutrient profile carbs-protein-fat (approx.)	Lead ingredients (based on label listing)	Comments/ explanations of words italicized in other columns
Awesome Mass Gainer 4000 (Horleys Health)	410	100	60-25-15	Maltodextrin, nonfat milk solids, dextrose, whey protein concentrate, coconut oil (*medium chain triglycerides*), fructose, yogurt powder, and creatine monohydrate	Made and distributed in New Zealand; go to the company Web site (**horleys.com**) for purchase information. For a discussion of medium chain triglycerides, see the text on page 120.
Big Whey (Next Nutrition)	173	42	10-70-20	Whey protein concentrate	If you buy a Next product, a key ingredient will always be whey. Directions on this gainer are a little different; users are urged to space out protein intake evenly over 5–6 meals/day to stay primed for new growth. Don't ignore carbs; they are important for muscle growth.
Gainers Fuel 1000 (Twinlab)	700 (with 16 oz. whole milk as suggested: 1,000)	193.6	83-17-0 (67-18-15)	Glucose polymers and glucose, BCAAs, and fructose	You can use the product with water or nonfat milk to reduce fat calories.

(continued)

115

Table 6.2 *(continued)*

Product (company)	Calories per serving (in water unless noted)	Serving size (gm)	Macronutrient profile carbs-protein-fat (approx.)	Lead ingredients (based on label listing)	Comments/ explanations of words italicized in other columns
Gainers Fuel 2500 (Twinlab)	2140 (serving is 3 scoops in 24 oz. milk, or you can use 16 oz. water)	603	90-9-1 (using water reduces the total calories and can change the profile)	Glucose polymers and glucose, BCAAs, and fructose	Building lean muscle depends a lot on weight workouts—calories alone won't do it.
Hardbody Gainer (MLO)	920	239	75-20-5	BCAAs, fructose, and glucose polymers	MLO recommends using 3 times/day rather than once a day. Be careful not to use as a substitute for food.
Heavyweight Gainer 900 (Champion Nutrition)	630	154	65-20-15	Whey protein concentrate and hydrolysate, egg albumen, *glycine*, fructose, maltodextrin, canola and safflower oils, and medium chain triglycerides	Glycine is an amino acid, essential for the biosynthesis of creatine phosphate, bile acids, and other amino acids. It helps improve glycogen storage.
Massive Whey Gainer (Ultimate Nutrition)	628	165	60-35-5	Whey protein concentrate, glucose polymers, and crystalline fructose	

Product					
EAS Myoplex Mass (EAS)	500	130	60-28-12	A blend of maltodextrin, sucrose, and dextrose; whey-protein concentrate; calcium caseinate; milk protein isolate; and taurine, l-glutamine, sodium caseinate, and egg albumen	Formulated for post-workout use. The theory behind adding taurine is that it might support protein metabolism and cell volumizing.
Muscle Milk (Cytosport)	348	75	15-38-47	Caseins and caseinates; whey concentrates, isolates, and peptides; bovine *colostrum* extract; a lipid complex containing canola oil and polyunsaturated long-chain vegetable oils; and maltodextrin	The company uses a protein formula designed to come close to ratios found in human mother's milk. This product has bovine colostrum, a
Nutrition N-Large II (Prolab)	620	152	60-30-10		

Table 6.2 *(continued)*

Product (company)	Calories per serving (in water unless noted)	Serving size (gm)	Macronutrient profile carbs-protein-fat (approx.)	Lead ingredients (based on label listing)	Comments/ explanations of words italicized in other columns
Progain (Biomax)	495	120	55-25-20	Maltodextrin, whey protein blend, and medium chain triglycerides	You may have to get this British product from a Web-based retailer.
Power Mass 1000 (Optimum Nutrition)	650	168	70-20-10	Whey protein concentrate and isolate, egg albumen, complex carbohydrates, and fructose	
Size Up Mass Gainer (Worldwide)	850	215	73-24-3	Amylopectins (complex carbs), glucose polymers, and whey protein concentrate and isolates	Contains a blend of ingredients often found in fat burners, such as guarana seed and kola nut; also contains some creatine and colostrum.
Super Heavyweight Gainer (Champion Nutrition)	900	200	48-22-30	Whey protein concentrate and hydrolysate, egg albumen, *glycine*, fructose, maltodextrin, canola and safflower oils, and medium chain triglycerides	

Product					
Super Mega Mass 2000 (Weider)	520	150 gm	78-20-2	Maltodextrin, corn syrup solids, nonfat dry milk, whey protein concentrate, crystalline fructose, dextrose, calcium caseinate, and egg albumen	
Vyo-Pro Whey Protein (AST Sports Science)	93	25 gm	13-77-10	Whey protein	
Whey Gainer (Better-Bodies)	378	100 gm	67-32-1	Maltodextrin, whey protein isolates, and fructose	May be difficult to get outside of Germany; check the Web.

supplier like Protein Factory **(www.proteinfactory.com),** you can customize your protein blend and select the flavors and sweeteners you wish to add. A look at the approximate prices of the different proteins gives you not only a sense of what you would have to spend if you created your own formulas but also some sense of the relative costs of the ingredients in commercially available products (see table 6.3).

In adding the carbohydrate component, you have lots of options, including whole food. For example, an eight-inch banana will give you 30 grams of carbohydrates; use a yellow one, not a ripe one, to stay within the moderate-GI range. For about $10, you can buy 500 milligrams of maltodextrin (glucose polymers derived from wheat) to take your caloric intake above maintenance requirements. As you can see on the weight gainers chart and on the energy bar chart (table 2.1), maltodextrin is a complex carbohydrate at the head of the ingredient list for many performance-enhancing products.

You can also purchase essential fatty acids independently and add them to your mix. Just remember that even though they are considered good fats, they still deliver the same number of calories as any other fat—nine per gram.

In the weight gainers chart, you also see several references to another kind of fat—medium chain triglycerides (MCTs). MCTs, which you can also buy independently and add to your program or formula, are saturated fats. They are considered useful in low-carbohydrate programs (also known as ketagenic programs) because they are more rapidly absorbed and burned as energy, so that they are associated with preworkout formulas. They can boost your energy levels when you

Table 6.3 Sources of Protein

Protein source (from least to most expensive)	Price per pound (in U.S. dollars)
Rice protein	$3.39
Soy protein isolate	$3.89
Whey protein concentrate	$4.25
Soy isolate XT (more isoflavones)	$4.89
Egg white protein	$5.00
Caseinate protein	$5.49
Milk protein isolate	$5.49
Ion exchange whey isolate	$8.09
Hydrolyzed whey protein (Hydro 520)	$9.99

experience low blood glucose levels from a lack of carbohydrates, because you process MCTs more like carbs than fat. Sounds good, but here's the irony: MCTs are found in coconut oil, palm kernel oil, and butter—all substances that, for health reasons, you've been warned against. Just be aware of the risks and restrictions of using MCTs, and keep these considerations in mind when you select products that contain MCTs:

- Don't use them if you have any kind of liver problem.
- Don't use them if you have a problem with your serum cholesterol level.
- Don't consume them on an empty stomach, or you may experience gastrointestinal upset.
- Don't use them in cooking.
- Initially, use only one tablespoon at a time until you know exactly how much you can take without upsetting your stomach.

Gaining Advantages Through Hormone Management

Anabolic steroids are the illegal shortcut to enhanced vascularity, stronger muscles, and a noticeable weight gain from increased lean mass. The legal shortcut in most countries (as of this writing) is a category of products called prohormones, which create the conditions for muscle building to occur. If you order products over the Internet or travel to different parts of the world be aware that several countries (including Australia, Canada, Germany, and the United Kingdom) restrict the purchase or use of prohormones.

When you understand a little about how the different prohormones and complementary products work in the body, you will see why companies try to sell you on *stacking*, or using multiple products together that contain hormone precursor substances and enhancers. On the surface, they may seem to duplicate functions, but in many cases they don't. For example, chrysin appears to minimize the conversion of testosterone to estrogen, a natural process called aromatization. For this reason, it is sometimes used in conjunction with a pro-hormone to get the maximum benefits of the testosterone-boosting supplement while mitigating the unpleasant side effects, such as bad skin and male-pattern baldness.

Scrupulous prohormone manufacturers offer their customers important warnings. The **netrition.com** Web site posts warnings like this one along with prohormone product descriptions:

Prohormones are not for use by children, teenagers, pregnant or nursing women. Do not use this product if you have breast, uterine, ovarian or prostate problems. If you are under medical supervision, consult with your physician before taking product. Too much testosterone before being fully grown could cause premature closure of the growth plates which control the growth of the body's long bones. This could stunt growth. Do not take prohormones until you have reached your full growth potential. Cycling Recommendations: We recommend that you take three weeks off for every six weeks of taking prohormones to prevent your body from adjusting to the exogenous (external) source of hormones. As always, consult your physician before taking any product that may alter hormone levels.

Here's another example:

Androgenic products should only be used by healthy males 21 years of age or older . . . People with any preexisting hormonal dependent cancers (i.e. prostate, breast, etc.) should avoid ALL andro products until more is known regarding the relationship of the testosterone precursors and the above afflictions. We recommend all people using any andro products get hormone testing done on a regular basis. We also recommend any man over 50 years old have a prostate exam and PSA to rule out the presence of microscopic cancer.

Netrition.com also offers some worthwhile guidance on dosages for all athletes: never take more than 600 milligrams of combined prohormones in one day. You want to support growth without risking your health, and inflated dosages will jeopardize your health.

Key terms used to describe the function of prohormone products include *anabolic, androgenic, cortisol blocking,* and *estrogen blocking*. The focus is on increasing hormone levels to accelerate muscular development and muting the body processes that interfere with that process or slow it down.

Testosterone is generally considered a male hormone, but ovaries also produce small amounts of it. Other hormones, called androgens, which are made in the ovaries and adrenal glands, have testosterone-like effects. Again, these hormones are not for men only. Androgens affect energy, sex drive, aggression, appetite, and muscle mass. While an excess of them in women will cause facial hair growth, acne, enlargement of the clitoris, deepening of the voice, and coarsening of the skin, a sufficiency will aid overall health and well-being.

DHEA and Human Growth Hormone

The first prohormone to gain mainstream popularity was DHEA (dehydroepiandrosterone), which athletes as well as middle-aged men and women used for years to engender some of the desirable "male-hormone" effects mentioned above—energy, sex drive, and muscle mass. Here is the science behind DHEA's effects in the form of a simple flow chart that shows a main pathway your body uses in the production of testosterone:

Cholesterol => Pregnenolone => **DHEA** => Androstenedione => Testosterone

Your adrenal glands make DHEA just before puberty. DHEA levels peak in your mid-20s and then go downhill, so if you are under 25, then your body is still making plenty of DHEA on its own. Studies suggest that DHEA increases Insulin Growth Factor 1 (IGF-1) levels and subdues the catabolic effects of cortisol.

IGF-1 belongs to a family of proteins that is important for normal human growth and development. For athletes, specifically bodybuilders, the mystique of IGF-1 relates to its supposed connection to lean-muscle building. Just as your body makes DHEA, it also manufactures IGF-1, but it makes less of it as you grow older. Human growth hormone (HGH), a hormone like testosterone, estrogen, and DHEA, is the ever-diminishing source. Produced and secreted by the pituitary gland, HGH is converted in the liver to IGF-1. Some products purport to boost the body's supply of HGH or IGF-1 directly; that is, they claim to provide the substance itself instead of simply creating the conditions whereby your body is stimulated to make it. Various IGF-1 studies, such as those reported by the department of neurology at Baylor College of Medicine (Lai et al. 1995) have shown that the substance must be administered by injection to be effective. The injection is given under the skin, the same way diabetics take insulin. A sublingual delivery system may give some results, but it is a huge step down in terms of value. Taking IGF-1 orally is pointless, because your stomach will digest it before it reaches your bloodstream.

Many of the prohormone products, not just DHEA, claim to blunt cortisol. Those claims can be a little misleading. Cortisol is not absolutely the enemy. Cortisol, or hydrocortisone, is a hormone of the adrenal gland and has important metabolic and anti-inflammatory effects. The primary reason why muscle builders fear it is that cortisol reduces the reserves of protein in all body cells except cells of the liver and gastrointestinal tract. In other words, it has a catabolic effect. Elevated cortisol levels also give rise to anxiety, panic attacks, and depression. On the other hand, low cortisol levels can lead to chronic fatigue.

Andro

On the flow chart that appears previously in this chapter, after DHEA comes the substance many people know as "andro." In 1996, OSMO's

Androstene 50 was the only Androstenedione product on the American market, and no one was talking about Norandrostenedione in the health food stores. Now, about 100 andro and norandro products are readily available without restrictions to athletes in American and other countries.

The positives of supplementation with these substances are explored below. First, here are the negatives. When an athlete takes too many testosterone precursors or androgens, the result may not just be a cosmetic nightmare. It can be what anabolic steroid users know as "roid rage"—short for "steroid rage." You can get too much of the prohormone products, so do not exceed recommended dosages unless you have a really savvy doctor by your side who is charting your physiological and psychological reactions to the supplements. When you add thermogenic ingredients to promote fat burning, such as ma huang and caffeine, some prohormone products can throw you into an anger that's unnatural—and scary to people around you. I can tell you from personal experience with a power-lifting friend: Overdosing on these hormone boosters can cause radical, violent behavior. Be sure you have good friends with you as you try a new product or an increased dosage.

Returning to the terminology, here are basic descriptions of the different substances that form the backbone of prohormone products:

• **Androstenedione** is a direct precursor of testosterone. It is produced in the adrenal gland, testes, and ovaries, and it is quickly converted into testosterone. To some extent, it is also converted to the so-called female hormones in men. Cholesterol figures into these conversion processes, so some labels emphasize how the products manage the conversion process by addressing the role of cholesterol.

• **Androstenediol** is in the same family as Androstenedione. Both are derived from DHEA, and both are converted to testosterone in the body. Manufacturers tout the advantages of Androstenediol by noting that your body converts it to testosterone more efficiently and that it isn't converted to estrogen.

• **Norandrostenedione** is converted not to testosterone but to a substance called nortestosterone, or nandrolone. Even though the difference between testosterone and nortestosterone is a minor structural one, that difference greatly enhances nortestosterone's anabolic properties. When testosterone and nortestosterone enter a cell, they bind to steroid receptors. Nortestosterone remains attached to these receptors longer than testosterone, yielding a more persistent anabolic effect. It also is not as readily converted to estrogen as testosterone is—the aromatization process mentioned earlier.

As table 6.4 shows, you will commonly see Androstenedione and Androstenediol preceded by the numeral 4 or 5. The first substance in

Table 6.4 The Prohormone Chart

Product (company)	Dosage	Lead prohormones and other active ingredients per dosage	Function(s)	Comments/ explanations of words italicized in other columns
3-Andro Xtreme (AST Sports Science)	2 capsules 30–45 min. before workout	4-Androstenediol (100 mg), 5-Androstenediol (100 mg), 19-Norandrostenedione (100 mg), caffeine (200 mg), and ephedra (400 mg)	Produces testosterone and nortestosterone; burns fat	Formula focuses on stimulating the central nervous system and boosting hormones.
5-Andro-Diol 100 (Human Development Technologies)	1 capsule 2 times/day	5-Androstene-3B, 17B-Diol (100 mg)	Boosts immune system and blocks cortisol and estrogen	
4-Diol 250 (AST Sports Science)	1 capsule 2 times/day	4-Androstenediol (250 mg)	Increases protein synthesis and muscle tissue recuperation	Note the differences in the characteristics assigned to 4-diol versus 5-diol, particularly the reference to immune system boosting—a function commonly assigned to 5-Androstenediol products.
5-Diol 250 (AST Sports Science)	1 capsule 2 times/day	5-Androstenediol (250 mg)	Produces testosterone, increases protein synthesis, and boosts immune system	

(continued)

Table 6.4 *(continued)*

Product (company)	Dosage	Lead prohormones and other active ingredients per dosage	Function(s)	Comments/ explanations of words italicized in other columns
7-Keto Fuel (Twinlab)	1 capsule daily	DHEA (3-Acetyl-7-Oxo-Dehydroepiandrosterone)	Blocks cortisol and increases testosterone-to-cortisol ratios	Natural levels of DHEA decline when people reach their 40s, so it usually has a greater impact on older athletes.
19-Nor 250 (AST Sports Science)	1 capsule 2 times/day	19-Norandrostenedione	Produces nortestosterone	
Andro Blast (Human Development Technologies)	2 capsules before workout	4-Androstene-3, 17-dione (500 mg), ma huang (300 mg), and caffeine (200 mg)	Produces testosterone, burns fat, and blocks cortisol	Formula focuses on stimulating the central nervous system and boosting hormones.
Androbolic (Kaizen)	2 tablets every 6 hr.	19-Norandrostenedione (100 mg), 4-Androstene-3, 17-diol (100 mg), 5-Androstene-3, 17-diol (50 mg), tribulus (250 mg), and chrysin (150 mg)	Supports androgenic growth	This product contains a coating that slows its breakdown, labeled a time-release complex. Your own stomach and digestive process can affect your level of absorption of a time-release product.

Androdiol (Genetic Evolutionary Nutrition [GEN] OSMO Therapy, Ergopharm, Sports One, and others)	[See the labels of the individual distributors]	4-Androstene-3beta,17beta-diol	Supports muscle growth and increases energy levels	Patrick Arnold developed the process to manufacture this chemical and holds a patent on its use. It is produced by his company, LPJ Research, and marketed by the companies listed.
Androdiol Heat (Ergopharm)	4 capsules a day before workout	4-Androstenediol (100 mg), caffeine (200 mg), and ephedra (20 mg)	Produces testosterone and burns fat	Formula focuses on stimulating the central nervous system and boosting hormones.
AndroPlex 700 (AST Sports Science)	2 capsules 2 times/day	Tribulus (500 mg), Androstenedione (100 mg), and DHEA (100 mg)	Produces testosterone	AST advises that this product, a stack of testosterone boosters, is not recommended for women because of its androgenic effects. It should also not be taken for more than 6 weeks straight.
Androsol Sports Skin Tonic (Biotest)	Spray it on; an 8-oz. (240-ml) bottle lasts 12–30 days	4-Androstenediol (50 mg/ml)	Produces testosterone	Topical application of pro-hormones was reportedly an early popular way of using them. The formula contains isopropyl (rubbing) alcohol; it can dry the skin or cause a rash.

(continued)

127

Table 6.4 (continued)

Product (company)	Dosage	Lead prohormones and other active ingredients per dosage	Function(s)	Comments/explanations of words italicized in other columns
Andrydyne (Cytodyne)	3 capsules	19-Norandrostenedione (100 mg), 5-Androstene-38, 178-diol (50 mg), and Androstenedione (4-Androstene 3, 17-dione; 50 mg)	Provides anabolic/androgenic support	This product puts three popular prohormones together in one package; it also contains chrysin.
Animal Stak (Universal)	1 pack/day	4-Androstendione (100 mg), 19 Nor-5-Androstenedione (50 mg), 5-Androstenediol (50 mg), DHEA (50 mg), large doses of amino acids, colustrum (250 mg), and *tribulus terrestris* (250 mg)	Produces testosterone, enhances growth hormone, and stimulates *luteinizing hormone* (LH)	This product is formulated for a 21-day cycle. Tribulus terrestris is a powerful herb that may increase levels of luteinizing hormone, which affects testosterone levels.
Cyclo-Bolic (Kaizen)	2 tablets before workout; taken sublingually	4-Androstenediol (25 mg), 19-Nor-4-Androstenedione (15 mg), 19-Nor-4-Androstenediol (8 mg), tribulus (250 mg), chrysin (50 mg), ma huang (25 mg), and caffeine (90 mg)	Produces testosterone, burns fat, and blocks cortisol	The manufacturer recommends sticking to a cycle of 6–8 weeks on the product, then 2 weeks off.
Di-Indolin (SportsOne/Klein)	1 capsule 3 times/day with food	Di-indolylmethane vitamin E phosphatidylcholine (300 mg)	Manages estrogen	This product is also called di-indolylmethane, or DIM.

hGH-PH Complex (Performance Bio Labs)	1 packet (14gm) mixed with 5 oz. water on an empty stomach at bedtime or before workout	4-Androstenediol (25 mg), 5-Androstenediol (25 mg), 1-Norandrostene (25 mg), 10-Norandrostene (25 mg)	Increases growth hormone production	Human growth hormone research is ongoing and worth following.
IsoDyne (Cytodyne)	1 capsule 3 times/day	5-Methyl-7-Melthoxy-Isoflavone (150 mg), 7-Isopropoxy *isoflavone* (150 mg), and Naringenin (50 mg)	Reduces cortisol and estrogen levels	The key here is isoflavones, water-soluble chemicals found in many plants. Research in the 1970s by the Hungarian company Chinoin yielded isoflavones without estrogenic effects and with anabolic value. (Soy isoflavones are recommended for aging women because of their estrogenic effect.)
Nortesten (MuscleTech)	2 capsules once a day	Norandrostenedione (36 mg), 19-Nor-4-Androstene-3, 17-Diol (36 mg)	Produces nortestosterone	This time-release product is not for women or men under 18.

(continued)

Table 6.4 *(continued)*

Product (company)	Dosage	Lead prohormones and other active ingredients per dosage	Function(s)	Comments/ explanations of words italicized in other columns
Paradeca (VPX Sports)	2 cc (oral syringe provided) 3 times/day	4 Androstenediol,19-Nor-4-Androstediol, and Androtriol (375 mg) combined	Produces nortestosterone and testosterone	The manufacturer offers some very specific recommendations about timing, including how long to hold the product in your mouth before swallowing it, length of the on- and off-cycles, and the number of hours between dosages.
Prolab Cyclo 4 Andriodiol (Prolab)	1 tablet daily; taken sublingually	4 Androstenediol (25 mg), beta cyclodextrin (86 mg)	Produces testosterone	Beta cyclodextrin is commonly used in sublingual prohormone products; this molecule appears to have the potential to allow lower dosages of the prohormone to be used to achieve the same effect as higher dosages. Don't swallow the product whole, however, or you will negate the advantages of the sublingual delivery system.

Product	Dosage	Ingredients	Effects	Notes
Pro-Male (Med-Lean)	Topically apply 1 ml of gel once daily for a month, and then decrease dosing to 1 ml just 4–5 times per week for 3 weeks each month	Androstenediol (30 mg), Norandrostenediol (15 mg), Norandrostenedione (15 mg), DHEA (10 mg), progesterone (5 mg)	Boosts androgenic and anabolic effects while minimizing side effects such as hair loss	Progesterone is included to act as an anti-estrogen; this is clearly not a product that female athletes should use.
Stenandiol (German American)	1 of each of 3 different products	#1: 4-Androstene 3, 17-dione (50 mg), and 5a Androstene-3B-17-Diol (50 mg) #2: 19-Nor-4-Androstenediol (50 mg) and 19-Nor-4-Androstenedione (50 mg) #3: Tribulus terrestris (500 mg)	#1: Produces androgenic growth #2: Produces anabolic growth #3: Stimulates LH (luteinizing hormone)	This product is a prepackaged stack, not a combination of different substances in one product, like many other products.

andro products was 4-Androstenedione, and, because of its estrogenic effects, the products containing it usually include anti-estrogen substances such as dihydroxyflavone or chrysin. In comparison, 5-Androstenedione works on different enzymes from its 4-dione cousin, but it is still associated with estrogenic effects. A more recent entry into the prohormone market, 4-Androstenediol, reportedly converts to testosterone faster than the diones, but research about its conversion rate to estrogen needs to continue. Empirical evidence suggests that the conversion to estrogen is not as fast as the conversion to testosterone, but, to safeguard the effectiveness of their diol products, manufacturers often combine anti-estrogen substances in them, too. In theory, you should be able to take lower dosages of 4-diol than dione, and the prices of several diol products are lower than the prices of their dione counterparts. Finally, 5-Androstenediol, which works slightly differently from 4-diol, appears to have more value in boosting the immune system than in testosterone production.

Because of the small structural difference between testosterone and nortestosterone, you will commonly see nortestosterone listed as 19-Norandrostenedione, which is the formal description of the molecule. 19-Norandrostenedione is a testosterone molecule that is missing a carbon atom in the 19th position and a hydrogen atom in the 17th position. When your liver processes it, a hydrogen atom is added in the 17th position, but the liver doesn't add the carbon atom in the 19th position. The result is a testosterone molecule missing that one carbon atom.

Nandrolone, or nortestosterone, is the base ingredient in Deca-Durabolin. Popularly known as Deca, it was one of the most popular steroids in the 1980s, a high time for steroid dealers. Deca sales boomed because the product worked and offered relatively few side effects compared to some of the other products—both reasons for the surge in popularity of norandro products nearly 20 years later.

The debate over whether or not an athlete who takes Norandrostenedione or other andro products is "natural" has raged for decades, shaped somewhat by prominent amateur athletic organizations. At first, the International Olympic Committee added DHEA to its list of banned substances, which included anabolic steroids, but left andro alone. The irony for athletes is that a drug test showing elevated testosterone levels wouldn't be able to tell if the cause was andro or steroid use. The NCAA bans a much more comprehensive list of anabolic agents, including anabolic steroids, all the andros and norandros, DHEA, testosterone 2, clenbuterol (an asthma treatment considered an aid to fat loss), and a host of related compounds—an all-encompassing term that covers substances that are part of the class by virtue of their pharmacological action or chemical structure.

Many athletes and organizations will consider you a "natural" athlete as long as the supplements you take do nothing more than upgrade your ability to produce testosterone or nandrolone. In contrast, Deca-Durabolin *is* nandrolone. You inject it and that's the end of the story. The distinction between substances that enhance your body's natural abilities to produce hormones and the direct delivery of hormones guided the development of this book, which aims at helping natural athletes.

A number of prohormone products package versions of two or three of these substances together in a "stack" to promote both testosterone and nandrolone production. Even with these powerful products, follow the dietary lead of top strength and bodybuilding athletes like Bryan Neese and Mohamad Moussawi: Eat a base diet of healthy, relatively low-fat food to support peak metabolic efficiency. In other words, don't expect the prohormone products to do all the work.

These Will do Harm—Without Doing Any Good

No matter how desperately you are searching for effective bodybuilding products, do not use insulin or 1,4-butanediol (BD) as performance-enhancing products.

Despite laboratory evidence that insulin does not stimulate protein synthesis in the body, some athletes cling to the myth that it does. Unless you are an insulin-dependent diabetic with a prescription for the substance, do not use it under any circumstances. Too much could kill you.

BD is an industrial solvent that should never be ingested, regardless of the claims you hear. Seizures and death may result. Courtesy of the Association of Poison Control Centers (Zvosec and Smith 2000), here is a list of BD-containing substances; they may be available for purchase on the Internet, but they should never be part of your performance-enhancing regimen: Zen, Serenity, SomatoPro, InnerG, NRG3, Enliven, Growth Hormone Release Extract (GHRE), Thunder Nectar, Weight Belt Cleaner, Rest-Q, X-12, Dormir, and Amino Flex. Additional names include Orange fX, Rush, Lemon fX Drop, Cherry fX Bomb, Borametz, Pine Needle Extract, Promusol, and BVM. The active ingredient of BD products may be listed as: tetramethylene glycol, Sucol B, 1,4-butylene glycol, butane-1, 4-diol, butylene glycol, and 1,4-tetramethylene glycol. Labels may say "this product does not contain GHB or 2(3) furnanone dihydro."

(Note: GHB, known as the "date-rape" drug, is a chemical cousin of butanediol.)

Trimming Fat Starts With Focusing on Fat

Even in the nutritional Dark Ages when I was a bodybuilder, my trainer didn't tell me to have no fat in my diet. His rule was, "No *added* fat." This was the 1980s, before strength and bodybuilding athletes got savvy about the positive metabolic effects of essential fatty acids—linoleic acid (an omega-6 fatty acid), arachidonic, and alpha lineolenic acid (an omega-3 fatty acid). All we knew was that a certain amount of fat was required to process fat-soluble vitamins (A, D, E, and K). We also made a grand assumption that any fish was good fish, and feel very smart for having embraced that belief now that it's common knowledge that cold-water fish such as salmon, herring, mackerel, sardines, and trout provide valuable omega-3 fatty acids. "No added fat" meant no fried foods, no butter on anything, and no processed foods (like brownies or cake) that had fat added to them—in short, it's what most of modern medicine would call a heart-healthy, anti-cancer diet.

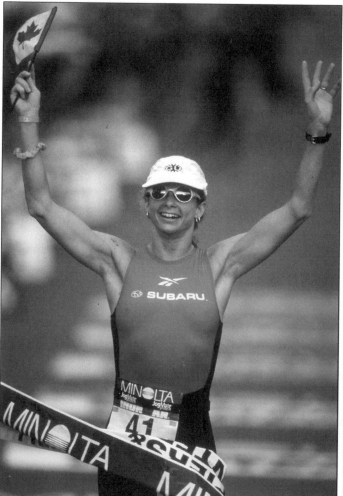

Lori Bowden added balance to her diet and the gold medal soon followed.

© Tom Putt/SportsChrome USA

The old-fashioned rule "no added fat," combined with a current understanding of how low-glycemic carbs versus high-glycemic carbs affect the body's metabolic responses, can lead directly to losing unwanted fat. Remember that high-GI carbs trigger a release of insulin (as explained in chapter 2), and there is plenty of evidence that high levels of insulin block the release of stored body fat as a source of energy.

Lori Bowden, one of the world's best Ironman triathletes, admits that she wanted to reduce her body fat when she first started shifting from simply running to doing triathlons at the age of 19: "When I first started in triathlon, I wanted to lose weight. We had to race in a bathing suit, so I was very conscious of how I looked." She effected the change through her basic diet, not through a reliance on fat burners or other supplements. The big change was moving away from a diet that centered on carbohydrates toward a diet that was relatively low in dietary fat but balanced in terms of carbs and proteins.

You may want to play with ratios eventually, but if you are new to the game of getting ripped for a bodybuilding show or needing to shed fat for other performance purposes, restructure your diet with a focus on fat. Avoid foods to which fat has been added. If you follow this suggestion, then you'll choose rice cakes as a snack instead of crackers and make your own soup out of defatted broth rather than eat soup out of a can. You'll also stay away from dairy products that contain fat.

Take a look at the kind of diet that elite bodybuilder Moe Moussawi sticks to in the weeks before a contest:

Sample On-Season Daily Menu to Cut Fat

Meal #1 (about 6:00 A.M.)

10 egg whites

1 baked potato

Calories in this meal total about 360, with 55 percent coming from carbs and 45 percent from protein. Unlike Moe's off-season breakfast, this one doesn't involve any fat that might be used to cook an omelet or give mashed potatoes a smooth consistency.

One hour later, at 7:00 A.M., Moe does weight training for one and one-half hours. Five minutes before the workout, he starts sipping Ultimate Orange, made by Next Nutrition.

A high-carbohydrate drink—62 percent carbs—with electrolytes and vitamin B6 to aid metabolism, Ultimate Orange also features thermogenic agents such as ma huang, caffeine, Korean ginseng, and cayenne pepper. Moe continues to sip it throughout his workout, which contrasts the way thermogenic aids in capsules are used—all at once at the beginning of the workout, with no ability to regulate ingestion. Moe says,

I have witnessed people going crazy after taking capsules. One guy in my gym took four capsules of [a product that is meant to be taken two capsules at a time], and he had a seizure. It was like planting a bomb in his stomach. At once, it exploded.

In capsule form, the athlete had ingested the equivalent of nine cups of coffee.

Meal #2 (immediately after the workout; about 8:30 A.M.)

Designer Protein shake (50 grams of protein)

10 grams glutamine

Meal #3 (about 10:30 A.M.)

16 ounces of chicken breast

steamed vegetables

Even chicken breast without skin contains fat, and in a serving this size, the fat grams total about eight, or 72 calories. A two-cup serving of vegetables provides about the same number of carbohydrate calories. The macronutrient distribution in this meal of about 360 calories is therefore 20-60-20.

Meal #4 (about 12:30 P.M.)

Designer Protein shake (50 grams of protein)

Meal #5 (about 2:30 P.M.)

8-ounce steak

1 baked potato

This meal involves no added fat, but it is not low-fat in the strict sense of the term. A lean, broiled porterhouse steak of this size offers 24 grams of fat along with 64 grams of protein. The potato provides 55 grams of carbohydrates, plus an additional 5 grams of protein. The macronutrient distribution in this 700-calorie meal is therefore 30-40-30.

Meal #6 (about 4:30 P.M.)

10 egg whites

About one and one-half hours later, at roughly 6:00 P.M., Moe does one hour of cardiorespiratory work, such as riding a stationary bike.

Meal #7 (immediately after the workout; about 7:30 P.M.)

Designer Protein shake (50 grams of protein)

10 grams glutamine

Meal #8 (about 9:30 P.M.)

1 can of tuna or a piece of salmon

Salmon and tuna provide both protein and omega-3 fatty acids, which are heart-healthy and help to burn fat. Nearly half the calories in a serving of salmon come from this type of fat. An essential fatty acid (EFA) supplement would be another way to introduce this nutrient to your diet.

Meal #9 (bedtime)

2 grams BCAAs

During the competitive season, Moe does not allow himself to go more than three and one-half hours without food. As a consequence, he gets up in the middle of the night for another protein meal.

Meal #10 (around 2:00 A.M.)

Designer Protein shake

Courtesy of Moe Moussawi, founder of Moe's Muscles

During the competitive season, Moe prepares no food with fat, reduces his carbohydrate intake, and reduces his overall caloric intake; those are the big changes from his off-season diet. This diet would not suit the performance needs of an endurance athlete, but it does show how one very successful bodybuilder integrates sports foods with a strict diet to sculpt his physique.

Fat Burners

Fat burners, or thermogenic aids, take advantage of the different ways that ephedrine, caffeine, and aspirin can play a role in reducing your body's fat stores, stimulating muscle growth, and making you feel energized. Ephedrine—the herbal form is ephedra—has been used for years to help counter obesity in adults, but it had a big performance problem: Its fat-burning effects diminished over time. Scientists looked at the whole interplay of chemical reactions and enzymes involved in breaking down fat for energy, and they realized that by adding caffeine and aspirin they could sustain ephedrine's fat-burning activity and even increase it over time.

Overuse makes thermogenic aids dangerous, so you have to be intelligent about using them. Even if they don't pose a threat to your health, these products could make you dangerous to someone else. You don't have to wander far on the Internet to read distressed admissions from high school football players about their road rage and brutal on-field behavior after ingesting these products. You might have lots of factors fueling explosive behavior—accelerated testosterone production, the excitement of a big game, rivalry with another athlete—so use good sense in introducing anything else that makes your system race.

The use of ephedra has even been linked to heart attacks, strokes, and seizures in a major study conducted by Neal Benowitz and Christine A. Haller at the University of California-San Francisco. Physician publications, such as *Anesthesiology News,* have also covered individual cases of people dying from combining stimulants or mixing them with prescription medicines.

Fat burners vary widely in price as well as in composition; the guidance in this chapter can help you avoid the enormous potential for being exploited. Sports products feature herbal stimulants such as those listed in table 6.5. Some are more powerful than others, because the amount of stimulant they deliver per milligram is greater.

Another herb that you'll often see among the list of ingredients is forskolin, derived from the root of coleus forskohili. It's not a stimulant; in fact, it's a medicine used to lower high blood pressure. It's also been linked to increased insulin secretion, which in turn regulates blood sugar level. Knowing this, you can see how it makes sense for a company to put

Table 6.5 Herbal Stimulants

Herb	Stimulant	Dose/serving of stimulant (approx.)	Cautions/ comments
Cayenne	Extract of the pepper		Extracts of this pepper can stimulate metabolism and provide other benefits.
Citrus aurantium (bitter orange extract)	Synephrine	Sports products commonly offer a standardized ratio of 16 mg of synephrine for 350 mg of herb	Research on synephrine is weak; it hints that this herb may not have as dramatic a metabolic effect as epheda, but also that it's not as potentially dangerous
Green tea	Caffeine	50 mg/cup	Green tea reportedly has benefits far beyond the caffeine, for example, strong antioxidant action.
Guarana seed extract	Caffeine	Sports products commonly offer a standardized ratio of 200 mg of caffeine for 910 mg of guarana	This herb contains compounds that slow the absorption of caffeine in the system, so it should deliver more sustained energy than coffee, for example.
Kola nut (bissy nut, cola)	Caffeine	200 mg is the common amount in sports formulas	None
Korean ginseng	Ginsenosides	Potency varies, but product should have 20–25 mg of ginsenosides for 500 mg of ginseng	This herb may possibly be effective in restoring muscle glycogen (*carbohydrate*) and high-energy phosphate compounds to normal levels.
Ma huang	Ephedra	Sports products commonly offer a standardized ratio of 20–25 mg of ephedra for 334 mg of ma huang	Don't take this herb while you're taking asthma medication or an antihistimine such as Sudafed.

Herb	Stimulant	Dose/serving of stimulant (approx.)	Cautions/ comments
Sida cordifolia	Ephedra	25 mg is common in sports formulas	In addition to acting like other sources of ephedra, this herb is used by Ayurveda physicians as an aphrodisiac; maybe you should avoid it if you don't want distractions during your workout!
White willow bark	Aspirin	Sports products commonly offer a standardized ratio of 15 mg of salicin (aspirin) for 100 mg of willow bark	People who have aspirin allergies want to stay away from this herb; definitely ask a doctor about taking it if you're on blood-thinning drugs, corticosteroids, or diabetes medication.
Yerba mate	Caffeine	50 mg is common	For centuries, natives in Africa and South America have ingested this herb to enhance sexual prowess, although its value here relates to its ability to raise body temperature and boost your adrena-line supply. Don't combine it with caffeine or antihistamines. Also avoid taking it with two amino acids found in many sports products, tyrosine and phenylala-nine, as well as cheese, chocolate, and beer.
Yohimbe bark (quebracho)	Extract of the bark	Sports products commonly offer a standardized ratio of 3 mg of stimulant for 100 mg of yohimbe	

it in a thermogenic product. On the other hand, you should generally avoid using forskolin if you're on an antihistamine.

To mitigate the dangers of using a thermogenic aid, follow these guidelines:

• Make your first dosage lower than the one recommended on the label, and take it with a meal to get a sense of how it affects you.

• Adjust your dosage to reflect your weight. It makes no sense that a 250-pound male bodybuilder would take the same amount of fat-burning product as a 110-pound female bodybuilder, yet many labels offer no guidance on adjusting the dosage. Cut the recommended dosage in half if you weigh less than 250 pounds—at least in the beginning.

• Adjust your dosage to reflect your lifestyle. If you indulge in coffee, cola, Mountain Dew, or other beverages with caffeine, you already pour a stimulant into your system. Compounding the effects with a thermogenic product inflates your risk of having a bad reaction.

• Don't take more than one thermogenic product at a time. This is easy to do inadvertently if you think of one product, like Red Bull or Ripped Force (American Body Building), as a preworkout energy drink, but you classify a product such as Xenadrine (Cytodyne Technologies) as a fat burner. Check the label of any product designed to get you into high gear, even an energy bar. Applied Nutrition's 151 Bar, for example, contains small amounts of Siberian and American ginseng root as well as cayenne.

• Try to find a liquid product that you like and that's affordable. You can sip a liquid fat burner/energy product so that the functional substances get into your system over time. Never gulp it, though, or you'll negate the advantages of having the stimulants in liquid form.

• If you take any prescription drugs, or if you've been taking over-the-counter decongestants or a headache remedy, do not use these products unless you check with a pharmacist or doctor—and not just any doctor will do. Find an internist who's an athlete, a sports medicine doctor, or an anesthesiologist. You want someone with a high awareness of drug interactions, particularly the interactions between the kind of stimulants you're using and other medications on the market.

Dropping Water Weight

The healthy and reliable way of dropping water weight starts with drinking water. In the weeks before your contest, make sure you are well hydrated so that your body doesn't get used to hanging on to water. In addition, during the week before your event, don't completely eliminate sodium from your diet—doing so would throw off your electrolyte balance, which is important for any athlete's performance—but do drop foods that naturally contain a lot of sodium. At this point, egg whites and canned tuna are no longer your best friends. Just two egg whites have more sodium (110 milligrams) than a four-ounce chicken breast (98 milligrams) or four ounces of white turkey meat (71 milligrams). A single can of tuna packed in water has 250 milligrams of sodium.

The day of your event is the time to turn down your water intake, but don't dehydrate yourself. If you're in a bodybuilding contest, the hot lights on stage and the demands of posing create the need for a certain amount of water and electrolytes to avoid cramping or fainting.

Regardless of whether you're a bodybuilder, a gymnast, or any other athlete who needs to keep water retention down, if you have dieted well, then you won't need to use diuretics. If you did not diet well, you still shouldn't be tempted to use diuretics, no matter what anyone tells you, who else uses them, or what the manufacturer claims. Diuretics are prescribed for people whose water retention places them at risk. An athlete who has prepared diligently for a contest does not fit in that category. Diuretics can tear up the physiology of normal, healthy people. Even athletes who thought they were knowledgeable and adept at using diuretics have had some rude awakenings, and—as in the tragic case of the early 1990s bodybuilding star, Momo Benaziza—the consequence

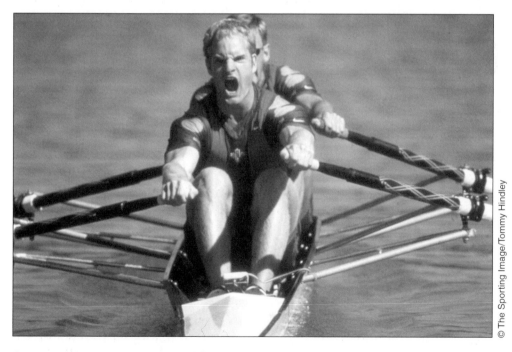

© The Sporting Image/Tommy Hindley

Some team sports require athletes to coordinate their weight very carefully so that team members match up well.

can even be death. What may have killed Momo is the extreme hypotension, or low blood flow, that resulted from a dramatic loss of electrolytes attributed to his diuretic use for the 1992 IFBB Grand Prix. His circulatory system simply failed. With all the excellent performance-enhancing supplements on the market to help you keep your system in balance while you cut fat and water weight, there is no reason to add your hypertensive mother's prescription diuretics to the mix.

Some people believe that dandelion root and leaves are safe and natural diuretics, but only weak clinical evidence supports the theory. In addition, dandelion causes skin reactions in some people, so go easy on the dosages if you decide to try this herbal approach. A typical dosage of dandelion root extract (5:1) is 250 milligrams three or four times a day.

Managing the Balancing Act

The desire to gain lean mass and cut fat, particularly if the goal is sculpting your body, can easily put your focus on products and practices that are potentially dangerous. This chapter covered many products that can help you safely accelerate the processes of building lean mass and trimming fat—but use them in dosages appropriate for the weight you are, not the weight you want to be. If your diet supports your appearance and performance goals, you will notice far more dramatic results than if you rely on the products alone.

CHAPTER 7

Handling Extreme Conditions

Extremes of temperature and altitude change the way your body responds to the food that you ingest. They can affect your desire to eat and even profoundly limit your ability to eat. Distance from convenient sources of food can also make an environment harsh—and make you look a lot like food to indigenous wildlife. Unusual stresses in a sport, such as the G-forces, are another factor that creates a severe environment and special nutritional needs.

Athletes who venture into harsh conditions are not the prime market for sports-food and supplement companies. Nearly all bars become too tough or brittle to eat in the cold and too mushy or sticky in extreme heat. The labels of protein powders often warn, "Do not expose to excessive heat, moisture, or sunlight" because the key ingredients lose their integrity under those conditions. On the other hand, a number of products happen to be well suited for extremes of heat, cold, altitude, dryness, or wetness, even though they weren't designed for use in those environments. Basically, athletes experiencing those conditions discovered through trial and error what worked, what didn't, and how to modify products to make them work. From dehydrated foods that cook with the sun's heat to gels that don't freeze to protein shakes that prevent muscle wasting at high altitudes, the industry has inadvertently produced a few products that perform well under demanding circumstances.

The Preparation Phase

Before these products even come into play during your adventure, you need to look at the specific ways the extreme activity will tax your body. Consider what body systems you will stress the most, and follow an eating and supplementation program to bolster those systems.

Heidi Howkins, who led international K2 expeditions from 1998 through 2000, as well as a 1999 Everest expedition, enriches her diet before a 25,000-foot climb with iron for her red blood cell supply and vitamin C for her immune system: "Three to five months prior, make sure available iron is as high as possible. You will deplete your hemoglobin on the mountain, so you have to build up in advance." She also recommends having hemoglobin levels measured during that period to ensure the desired effect.

Regardless of your sport, if you plan to subject your body to extreme stresses, you need supplementation that boosts your immune system. You also need to know precisely how your body reacts to the supplements under those extreme stresses. EAS used these starting points in designing a nutrition program for a top NASCAR driver, who often tackles back-to-back races Saturday and Sunday as a driver in both the Winston Cup and Busch series.

The specific program objectives were these:

- Strengthen the immune system to keep the athlete in optimum health

- Increase lean muscle mass to protect him in the event of impact

- Reduce body fat slightly to support a higher level of athleticism, but not drop it so low as to lose the protection that fat provides to joints and organs

- Increase protection for the joints

- Support a strong metabolic response to intense exercise in areas such as hormone production, muscle-tissue repair, insulin metabolism, and fat burning

- Enhance the body's ability to minimize muscle breakdown, build muscle, and decrease body fat

The program had to be structured for convenience so that the athlete could adhere to it despite a rigorous travel schedule. The NASCAR season is longer than the season for any other professional sport, with the drivers and crews traveling 38 weeks of the year. This particular athlete is on the road from Wednesday through Sunday, either flying or driving. The supplements he needed had to be with him at home, on the plane, or in a hotel, and they had to be worked into his schedule conveniently. There is a lesson in this for every athlete: Consider your lifestyle, habits, and time constraints when you create a nutritional program so that you can follow it consistently. You can't expect products that are designed to yield long-term benefits to boost your performance if you take them erratically. This lesson is particularly important if your undertaking places you in a high-risk environment like a racecar or the Sahara Desert.

To achieve the program objectives, EAS selected just a handful of supplements and one meal replacement to enhance this athlete's daily diet:

• Vitamin C, 1000 milligrams. Vitamin C is involved in forming collagen, a protein-based substance essential for healthy bones, teeth, skin, and tendons. It is also critical to immune function, supporting the healing of wounds and resistance to infection. Proper iron absorption depends on the presence of vitamin C, as does your body's metabolism of some amino acids and folic acid. These are just the highlights of its role in keeping your body sound. The RDA for an adult male or female 25 to 50 years old is a measly 60 milligrams, and the inherent shortcoming in this recommendation is that it does not reflect the extraordinary additional needs of athletes—particularly athletes in extreme situations. Both environmental and physical stresses place huge additional burdens on the body and inflate an athlete's need for vitamin C, which is why the dosage for a racecar driver is one gram. Athletes who routinely drink freshly squeezed juices and/or eat lots of fresh fruits and vegetables should not have a need for this level of supplementation.

• Two Myoplex shakes. The shakes are a simple way to add whey protein, which supports muscle development and resistance to infection. They also contain essential vitamins and complex carbohydrates. The athlete drinks one after his morning workout and one in the middle of the afternoon.

• Structured EFA, two capsules three times a day with meals. This standard amount helps any athlete ensure healthy levels of omega-3, omega-6, and other essential fatty acids, which optimize metabolic functioning. A less expensive and equally effective alternative is adding flaxseed oil to a shake.

• HMB, four capsules three times a day with meals. This supplementation allegedly enhances the body's own supply of hydroxy beta-methylbutyrate monohydrate (HMB) to help reduce muscle tissue breakdown.

• Glucosamine HCL, one capsule three times a day between meals. Like HMB, glucosamine occurs naturally in the body. It's a primary building block of the substances that make up cartilage and synovial fluid. Your body needs it for healthy joint function and especially appreciates an added dosage if you've inflicted damage on your joints.

• AAB (Athletes' Antioxidant Blend), one capsule three times a day. As noted previously in the discussion of vitamin C, high-stress environments intensify the body's need for certain nutrients. This is very true for antioxidants, which include vitamins C and E, beta-carotene, phytochemicals, and several other substances. These substances do not all function identically in the body, however, so a blend such as this offers a spectrum of benefits in a single supplement.

Courtesy of Rob Fulcomer, EAS, Inc., Golden, Colorado.

The athlete adopted this program during his race season, which included numerous personal appearances and media events in addition to the race-related travel. Within two months of starting it, the driver achieved his body composition goal: His body fat dropped from 14 to 10 percent. He also felt more vigorous and improved his strength and recovery time.

The real proof was in the driver's feeling of resilience during and after one of the greatest short-track events in America. On a half-mile, high-banked oval in Tennessee, drivers endure tremendous forces as they round the track. It is one of the most physically demanding scenarios: Cars in very close proximity collide and "tap" at speeds of 180 miles an hour or more, and powerful G-forces affect the drivers. Crediting the program, the athlete volunteered after the race that he felt the best he ever had. The taps and forces didn't bother him nearly as much as they had before.

On the Water

Although the length of their loop differs markedly from that of the NASCAR driver—the circumference of the globe rather than a half mile—crews of the Whitbread Round the World Race have many of the same requirements. The problem is, they may include supplements and other performance-enhancing products in their preparation, but they have difficulty integrating many of them into their eight months of travel from port to port. Nevertheless, they do rely heavily on one kind of food designed for athletes.

The Whitbread race has attracted top sailing teams from different nations since 1973. The choice of food and the amount of water brought on board has always reflected an obsession with weight. Like high-altitude mountaineers attempting to reach the summit of Everest or K2, the Whitbread racers cut the handles off their toothbrushes to reduce the amount of weight they must carry. On board, they may have eight titanium spoons for a crew of 12. They have also been known to jettison food to improve boat speed. (Similarly, I've seen adventure racers bury food and supplies they decided they didn't need to accelerate their pace during an Eco-Challenge.) Through rigorous training and dieting, the Whitbread racers also tend to reduce their own weight by dropping body fat. According to Dr. Reynaldo (Rudi) Rodriguez, who shared his experience online when he served as physician for the American and Norwegian teams during the seventh Whitbread, body fat compositions of 8 to 9 percent are common prior to the start of the race. Nutrition is a vital concern during this race so that they don't drop below those levels. The crews carefully plan what food comes aboard. In his notes posted on *The Physician and Sportsmedicine Online* Web site listed in the Selected Resources section of this book, Dr. Rodriguez notes that the sailors have science behind their choices:

> Swedish research during the 1993–1994 racing season established that calorie requirements for Whitbread sailors are between 4,500 and 5,000 calories per crew member. Each team has devised its own program with different calorie intakes and vitamin and mineral supplements. Nutritionists, dietitians, and physicians have been involved in the planning for each team. Olive oil has gained almost uniform acceptance as a dietary staple due to its high calorie density, its taste when added to freeze dried food, and its apparent ability to aid GI transit. Food may be rationed, the sailors may complain about it, but it is rarely thrown overboard any longer.

Over the years, technology has developed to help the sailors dramatically reduce the weight of their supplies without endangering their health. Racers carry very little water. They depend on reverse-osmosis water makers powered by diesel engines, because hand-powered emergency water makers can't provide enough water for their basic needs. With plenty of freeze-dried food on board—Dr. Rodriguez says it now "is universally used during this race"—the crews can remain well fed the entire time. That is, unless the technology fails. During the seventh Whitbread, which began in Southampton on September 21, 1997, that's what happened.

> *Dehydration.* While traumatic injuries were uncommon, technical problems with water makers on Swedish Match and Chessie [Racing, of the United States] caused both crews to ration water and collect rainwater. (Cold weather conditions can cause the water makers to malfunction.) Swedish Match seemed to suffer the most. The crew was restricted to 2 to $2\frac{1}{2}$ cups of water a day for [two] weeks. Complaints of dizziness, thirst, lethargy, and myalgia were common. However, the marked weakness and loss of efficiency while racing was considered the biggest problem.

> Fortunately, as water and ambient temperature increased toward the end of leg 5, water production increased also. . . . On board Chessie, the situation was not quite so grim. They were able to

repair their water maker after receiving parts from the U.S. delivered off the coast of Cape Horn during an emergency stop.

Inadequate nutrition was also a concern for both boats. Without water to rehydrate the freeze-dried provisions, the crews were reduced to eating dry cereal, olive oil, candy bars, and other non-freeze-dried foods. Body fat compositions of 8 percent to 9 percent were common prior to the start of the race and still, several of the sailors lost more than 6 kilograms of weight. Weakness remained a problem for many to the finish (Rodriguez 1998).

Freeze-Dried Meals: Food for Land, Water, and Space

Freeze-drying and dehydration do create remarkably light, nutritious products, and they certainly tend to hold more gustatory appeal than MREs. For readers not familiar with this U.S. military designation, MREs are relatively heavy, plastic-encased collections of little boxes of calorie-dense foods that many soldiers have probably wanted to give to the enemy. Depending on how you feel at the moment, the acronym either means "Meals Ready to Eat" or "Meals Refusing to Exit."

Freeze-drying fresh or cooked foods—grains, beans, fruits, meats, seafood, pastas, vegetables, and eggs—begins the same way that frozen foods are made, but it involves multiple other steps that make the foods suitable for athletes on extended adventures. After the foods are flash frozen, they are put in vacuum chambers that are as cold as negative 50 degrees Fahrenheit and then subjected to a heat method that turns the ice into a gas without melting it first. Through the freeze-drying process, the manufacturer ultimately removes about 98 percent of the product's moisture, which prevents the food from spoiling. Special packaging that serves as a barrier to moisture and oxygen helps give the food a very long shelf life.

The difference between frozen and freeze-dried food is obvious—you have to keep frozen food frozen until you use it, or it will lose its integrity. The difference between dehydrated and freeze-dried food is less obvious, however, because both of them are shelf stable. One difference that could be important to competing athletes is that freeze-dried foods reconstitute at a somewhat faster rate. On the other hand, many athletes who use this kind of food on the trail (or on the boat) don't take the time to wait around while the water reconstitutes the food. They pour the water in the bag, roll up the bag, and stuff it back in their pack while they keep racing. Later, when they reach a stopping point or slow-down in the event, they pull out the bag and have dinner.

Aside from price—you can expect to pay as much as $7 for some freeze-dried foods—one potential downside of these products is pack volume. While these foods are light, they take up a lot of space compared to a bar. You won't find top Eco-Challenge competitors willing to indulge in the relatively fine dining afforded by freeze-dried foods when they have to make room for climbing gear and wet suits in their backpacks. You can transfer the foods into smaller plastic bags, but this is not a desirable option if your race involves moving through water.

No Soup, but Plenty of Nuts

For events like an eight- or nine-day Elf Authentic Adventure or Eco-Challenge, many performance-enhancing products could support an athlete's needs, but many of the best racers opt not to rely on them heavily. For example, Lisa Smith, an elite ultra-runner and multisport adventure racer, combined science with trial and error to come up with remarkably simple nutrition plans for the different long-distance training sessions and events she does in harsh conditions. She backs up an astonishing list of endurance accomplishments with a masters degree in health education and fitness, 15 years of experience as a personal trainer, and advice from biochemist Dr. Nick Abrishamian.

Lisa's nutritional challenges are not only to meet high caloric requirements, but also to minimize the ravages of extreme temperatures. Her events include contests like these:

- Five Badwater 135 ultramarathons (from Death Valley to Mt. Whitney)
- Two Marathon de Sables ultramarathons (a 145-mile, self-sufficient desert run in the Moroccan Sahara; in 1999, Lisa became the first American, male or female, to win the event in its 15 year history)
- GNC National 100k championship (Pittsburgh, March 2000; Lisa was on the first-place team, placed first among female runners aged 30 to 39, and placed seventh among all female runners)
- World 100k team championship (France, 1999; Team USA)
- Seven Hawaiian Ironman championships
- World duathlon and triathlon championships
- Three Eco-Challenge multisport adventure races
- Two Raid Gauloises multisport adventure races
- Two ESPN X Games multisport adventure races
- 17 ultramarathons (50 miles or more)
- More than 90 marathons (with a personal record of 2:48:52)

At first, Lisa's nutritional challenge for these events was compounded by a medical condition:

> I had a thyroid problem that would be so, so insignificant to people who aren't exercising. But I was passing out in the pool. I went to a specialist in Houston, Texas, who diagnosed a thyroid problem. I was getting ready for the Ironman in New Zealand, and he said, "There's no way you'll make it through." It was a minor problem, but for someone who was competing at this level, it was a major problem.

For a time, she did take prescribed medication and felt it helped. In the long run, she credits Nick Abrishamian with putting her back on track. After exhaustive blood tests to determine her individual needs, he formulated Lisa-specific supplements, including a protein powder that she puts in the food she takes on races. She firmly believes in eating for your blood type, and hers (O+) requires high protein. As a result, her winning run in the Marathon de Sables—the 145-mile "Marathon of Sand" in the Sahara Desert—was fueled by Nick's powder, which she put in packages of Mountain House freeze-dried foods and complemented with nuts.

> You are responsible for carrying everything for [seven] days— breakfast, lunch, dinner, [and] snacks—and you have to have at least 2,000 calories. And the race organizers allot you [nine] liters of water a day. So, scientifically, with my friend Dr. Abrishamian, I needed to figure this out. Two thousand calories is not a lot of food for someone running 50 miles a day. It's very cold at night— in the Sahara, it can get to 30 degrees [Fahrenheit]—and 120 or 130 during the day.

> It's all about what you're eating that's going to get you through the next day. I went to the store and searched and searched. I couldn't believe the high calories and protein in nuts. It looked like you had a little food, but you had a lot of food. People would look at me with my one bag of nuts and say: "That's all you have!" I'd say, "Yeah." I was taking 5,000 calories a day. I had a bunch of nuts all mixed together and I would suck on one nut at a time. Savored each little nut. The other thing I took was Mountain House [freeze-dried food]. I opened up the bag before the race and put it in large plastic baggies—it took up less room—and put [two] teaspoons of salt in each meal plus [three or four] scoops of Dr. A's protein powder. I discovered once I put it in these baggies, I could dump my water in them, set them out in the sun, and let them heat up

during the day. Then at the end of the day, I didn't need an oven or stove or matches that other people were using for their meals.

The next year, everyone I went with had the same system. . . . It's all about the food. It doesn't matter how long the race is, it's all about what you're going to eat.

Nuts and nut products belong in the packs of athletes undertaking a week-long foot race like the Marathon de Sables or a multisport expedition race like the Elf Authentic Adventure or Eco-Challenge, which can take as much as two weeks to complete. (The obvious exception is athletes with nut allergies.) Cathy Sassin, one of the world's best adventure racers, brings almond paste as well as bags of nuts on her treks.

The reason you get so many calories in such a little package is that about 75 percent of a nut's calories come from fat. Most nuts have

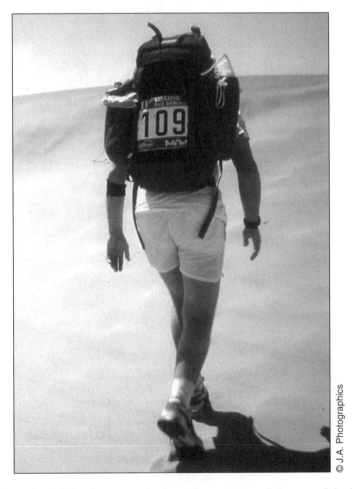

© J.A. Photographics

The Marathon de Sables is a good place for nuts and freeze-dried foods.

monounsaturated fat, but about two-thirds of the fat in walnuts is essential fats such as omega-3, the type found in fish. Protein supplies many of the remaining calories in many nuts; when you combine them with a whole-grain product, you get a meal with all the essential amino acids. In other words, peanut butter sandwiches are not junk food. Nuts also contain fiber, vitamin E, folic acid, niacin, vitamin B6, zinc, copper, magnesium, and valuable phytochemicals.

When Lisa's two friends from Morocco, former Marathon de Sables top finishers, were in the United States for the New York Marathon—they are 2:15 marathoners—they surprised many other athletes with their simple diet that, of course, included nuts. The only "supplement" they had ever used to prepare for the world's harshest foot race was green tea, which is known for its antioxidant properties. Their staple diet was couscous, a lamb-chicken stew, nuts, figs, and dates. Lisa did add an electrolyte drink (Cytomax by Cytosport) to their program, which gave them immediate positive results.

Eating Like the Natives

The experience of athletes like Lisa Smith and her Moroccan friends points to the central role that whole foods play during and after stressful athletic challenges. As a corollary, you can learn a lot about eating for extreme conditions from the indigenous people of an area. That doesn't necessarily mean you should eat precisely what they eat, but it does mean that you should choose performance-enhancing foods that feature the same nutrients.

Professional adventure photographer and athlete Michael Powers, who has helped lead kayaking and trekking trips in some of the most severe conditions on the planet, studies the habits and foods of indigenous peoples before he goes on his trips. For example, Michael explains that

> Indians used to talk about how they would get sick in the winter from eating animals that were too skinny. They would get ill from not having enough fat in their diet. It's apparent that when you're in cold climates, you need that fat.

If you are consistently taking on adventures in cold climates or water, then you should make sure your body fat levels support your energy needs in those conditions. You will need more dietary fat than athletes who seldom venture into frigid temperatures. If you're in the group that only occasionally takes on the cold, don't try to boost your body fat level dramatically for your event. In preparation for something like the Iditabike Extreme, in which cyclists race part of the Iditarod Trail before the dogs

A Comparison of One-Ounce Servings of Dried Nuts and Nut Products

Dried nuts don't contain much sodium, but commercially salted nuts contain 200 or 300 milligrams of sodium per one-ounce serving. The nature of your activity and climate affect the amount of additional sodium you need, which will determine whether you want to go with salted nuts or mix salted and unsalted nuts. See table 7.1 for a comparison of one-ounce servings of dried nuts and nut products.

Table 7.1   Nut Comparison

	Calories	Carbs (gm)	Protein (gm)	Fat (gm)
Almonds (20–24 nuts)	167	5.8	5.7	14.8
Almond butter	184	6.0	5.0	16.0
Almond paste	127	12.4	3.4	7.2
Brazil nuts (6–8 nuts)	186	3.6	4.1	18.8
Cashews (18 nuts)	163	9.3	4.4	13.2
Cashew butter	165	9.0	4.0	14.0
Hazelnuts (aka Filberts; 12 nuts)	179	4.4	3.7	17.8
Hazelnut butter	188	5.0	4.0	19.0
Macadamia nuts (12 nuts)	199	3.9	2.4	20.9
Peanuts (35 pieces)	160	2.5	7.0	13.5
Peanut butter (Brands can vary.)	190	5.0	9.0	16.0
Pecans (15 halves)	190	4.0	3.0	20.0
Pistachios (47 nuts)	164	7.1	5.8	13.7
Walnuts (14 halves)	190	3.0	4.0	18.0

Data from *The Complete Nutrition Counter* by Lynn Sonberg, 1993.

get there for the season, don't expect to make any short-term adaptations to the cold. Your main concerns for the 100-mile, week-long event will be wearing gear that protects you from wind and cold and keeping your water and food from freezing. You will be better served by a liquid meal replacement than by lots of additional dietary fat.

Michael does bring some of his own food supplies, but he tries as much as possible to eat the foods of the areas he visits. In some cases, it's an innocent adventure that gives him a chance to sample something unique and enjoy sources of nutrients that keep the natives healthy:

> When I got off the train that was taking us up to Machu Picchu, at the train station was a Quechua Indian woman dressed in her native garb. She had a big basket that was full of hot, steamed blue corn. This blue corn grows up there at 10 or 12 thousand feet and it's totally different from the corn that grows at sea level. It's wonderful. When you bite into it, you taste the earth of high-altitude Peru.

Michael's eating adventures don't always have such a poetic twist, however. When he was kayaking with a group of local paddlers in Bodô (pronounced "Buddha"), Norway, which is north of the arctic circle, he camped and ate with them. In this case, they had what they occasionally ate during a hard trip: whale stew. A hardy meal made from the minke whale—a type of small whale that is plentiful in the arctic water—the stew is not an aberration in Norway. Nor is it common. Norwegians in this area do not hunt the whales commercially; they do it solely for local consumption. For the hard-working, adventuresome people in the area, minke whale is "food for athletes." Back home in California, however, Michael's photos of a steaming cauldron of whale stew over an open fire drew fierce criticism—indigestion long after the fact.

On his trips to Antarctica, Everest, the Altiplano, and countless other demanding stretches of wilderness, Michael also brings his own food supplies, including different brands of energy bars that he'll toss into a dry bag stored in the kayak. More often, though, he brings his own sustained-energy convenience food called Michael's Magic Muesli, a nutritious mixture made out of the following ingredients:

- Organic rolled baby oats (baby oats are small particles that mix easily)
- Oat bran
- Raisins
- Nuts
- Unsweetened carob
- Dried papaya
- Soy powder
- Spirulina

The mix is truly very tasty and has high entertainment value: When you add a little apple juice or water, it turns green.

Special Needs, Special Foods

There are many environments where even Michael's muesli cannot work magic for athletes, though. For high-altitude mountaineers, there is essentially only one sport food that makes it to the summit. Heidi Howkins has said that energy gels are a staple of summit bids because they don't freeze above 26,000 feet. She says that she has also tried sweetened condensed milk: "At really extreme altitudes, you can't eat anything that will draw moisture from your stomach, because it will make you feel queasy." This is the primary value of energy gels, aside from the fact that they remain viscous without forming solid lumps. Because climbers can often get them down without feeling sick despite their intense aversion to consuming anything at that altitude, the gels do the most important thing a food can do—feed the brain. A squirt of energy gel can give the brain the sugar it needs to take the body to the top. This key to staying alert and healthy during a high-altitude climb builds on Heidi's pre-climb regimen of vitamin C and iron, described earlier in this chapter.

At high altitudes, climbers have no access to fresh produce, and even at base camp, protein can be hard to get. The camps have no refrigeration, but they are subject to a great deal of daytime heat on the glacier. Temperatures fluctuate wildly. Normally, climbers don't directly see how this affects their base-camp food supply, but on Heidi's 1998 K2 expedition, a helicopter had to take the ailing cook off the mountain, so the climbers cooked for themselves for a few days. As Heidi remembers,

> We developed a profound appreciation for the number of ways that eggs can go bad—gray ones, fluorescent green ones. We discovered the cook wasn't as careful as we were about picking the good ones. Here's a risk on the mountain we hadn't expected: salmonella.

A completely different set of concerns faces athletes who begin their high-altitude adventure at the top and head to sea level. Specifically, what food do you bring when you are about to skydive to the north pole?

When world-record skydiver Jim McCormick made the jump as part of an international expedition in 1995, he and his fellow jumpers knew that they could possibly be stranded at the pole after they left the Russian jet transport. They had to carry enough food and water to survive at least a few days—and anything they carried would have to fit under or into the polar suits they would wear underneath the backpacks with their parachutes.

Because the north pole has very dry air in addition to the frigid temperatures, the skydivers needed lots of water. Jim brought a Camelback system so that his water supply would stay flat against his body in

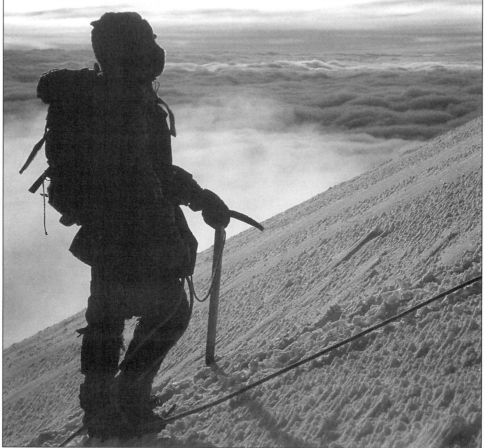

Energy gels can make it to the summit and remain edible, unlike other sports foods.

a bladder during the skydive; this approach would keep the water from freezing and protect the system from rupturing. Unfortunately, he couldn't wear the system the way it was designed to be worn, on his back. Putting it there would make it vulnerable to damage; moreover, if it were damaged, it would send water into his parachute gear, his primary survival system. Jim wore the Camelback in the front and put a specially designed insulating sleeve over the feed tube to prevent water in the tube from freezing.

He stuffed packets of trail mix—mostly nuts and dried fruit—into his polar suit, along with beef jerky for protein and salt. He scrupulously avoided anything with caffeine, realizing that a stimulant might force him to use the exit hatch on his polar suit. He also packed some energy bars. That move, he realized just before he exited the aircraft, was not a particularly good one. Energy bars of all kinds are inedible in freezing temperatures. All he could do was put them close to his body in an attempt to keep them malleable.

Fortunately, he didn't have to worry about that. The Russian support team picked up the skydivers in MI-8 helicopters shortly after they landed. They stopped first at an ice station and then went directly back to Siberia for reindeer and noodles.

Extreme Recovery

Extreme endurance athletes of all kinds—from ultramarathoners who race in the desert to high-altitude mountaineers on K2—put their bodies through amazing stress, even when they have a sound nutritional program. According to Dr. Bill Misner, who has studied nutritional needs of the Marathon de Sables racers, an average runner's estimated calorie burn during the seven-day race is at least 15,000. Bill breaks down the calorie sources as follows: 9,000 calories from body fat stores (that's nearly 2.5 pounds of body fat); 4,500 from muscle and liver glycogen stores (1.33 pounds); and 1,500 from amino acid pools in lean muscle mass (nearly .5 pounds of muscle). Daily fluctuations in water weight can also be profound, ranging from 5 to 12 pounds.

The recovery from such an ordeal is understandably daunting and must actually begin while the athletes are still racing. They continually try to replace lost electrolytes and aggressively try to replace lost calories at the end of the day. In general, they can do a good enough job to keep going. Through eating and drinking, they can restore an estimated 70 to 85 percent of fat stores, muscle glycogen, fluid levels, and electrolytes in the rest periods between stages. Bill, who is the head of research and product development for E-Caps Hammer Nutrition and a two-time former U.S.A. 50-Mile National Masters champion, says that there are some things the ultramarathoners can't replace. As he explained in an article for American Fitness Professionals and Associates,

> Complete lean muscle mass amino acid resynthesis and several micro-metabolites are not completely restored, tending to specific store depletion proportionate to duration, distance and/or intensity. It has been suggested that one day of rest is required for each mile raced for complete cyclic recovery prior to full-course training. Whoa, that is 145 days or so!

> Perhaps not quite that long, since each stage imposes a daily mandatory "rest" break, a divisive factor of 2 lowers the 145 day figure to 72.5 days, assuming each runner does not return to arduous training prematurely before down-deep cellular recovery is complete (Misner 2000).

Bill's nutritional guidelines for enhancing recovery after extreme endurance events, particularly those in harsh environments, are worth mentioning as a specific complement to the more general recovery information in chapter 3. He suggests following these five rules:

1. Ingest 1.4 to 1.7 grams of complete proteins per kilogram of bodyweight (about .75 grams per pound) throughout the recovery period.

2. Supplement your diet with either 2,000 grams of glutamine or 2,400 grams of APGL (arginine-pyroglutamate-lysine) per day, taken on an empty stomach. Evidence suggests that these supplements may enhance the release of human growth hormone.

3. Eat fiber to help eliminate toxins. You may take it in a supplement or get it from raw fruits and vegetables. However you do it, Bill recommends 35 to 60 grams per day with 100 to 120 fluid ounces of distilled water; raw fruit juices may enhance the process.

4. Include antioxidants in your regimen, at least in the 30 to 40 days after the race. The Moroccan runners relied on green tea, a great source of antioxidants. Other antioxidants include alpha-lipoic acid, vitamins C and E, gingko biloba, glutathione, and N-acetyl cysteine.

5. Avoid foods that impede your recovery, including anything with refined sugar, bleached flour, or other nutrient-robbing processing. Your rate of recovery will increase when most of your weekly dietary choices are whole raw fruits, vegetables, whole grains, nuts, legumes, seeds, and organic cereals, and when you take in either small or no amounts of alcohol, dairy byproducts, red meat, poultry, high-sodium foods, and diet products, including all high-phosphorus carbonated beverages.

CHAPTER 8

Fueling to Suit Your Age

If you could combine the physiological advantages of being a child with the timing, skills, and well-developed muscles of a disciplined adult athlete, you would be a formidable competitor—right? Well, to some extent, you can do that by choosing the right supplements. Even if you're in your late teens, if you want to win in your sport, you want to regain some of the advantages you had as a kid.

From the time male athletes hit their early 20s, they are in a steady state of decline. The window of optimal performance for female athletes may be a bit larger, but not much. Changes in your hormone production, endocrine system, nutrient absorption and retention, and levels of micronutrients decrease your ability to train intensely, recover from injuries, build muscle, and react quickly. Don't kid yourself by thinking that diligent training and a balanced diet of foods you buy at the grocery store are enough to counter the degenerative effects of aging. Unless you are fortunate enough to eat fruit right off the tree and juice organic vegetables grown in nutrient-rich soil, you may need supplements.

Supplements for Young Athletes

Performance-related supplement programs for athletes in their teens and 20s correlate to the competition's level of fitness and drive. At the X Games, for example, your competition most likely has a diligent training program but a fairly casual nutritional program. At the Olympics, you face athletes who are equipped with every advantage their countries and coaches can provide—and who are under a great deal of scrutiny about their dietary regimen.

For a book called *Lessons from the Edge,* which featured tips from extreme athletes, I interviewed young skateboarders, stunt bikers, and inline skaters, among others, about their training and eating habits. It wasn't uncommon for them to tell me that they relied on pizza on training days and a caffeinated energy drink like Red Bull during competition. At the age of 17 or 21, they didn't really care about a balanced diet, and their lack of discipline had no apparent impact on their performance.

Drinks With a Kick

More than any other sports foods, energy drinks spiked with caffeine or a similar stimulant are promoted to the active youth market as the number one source for a performance edge. As a consequence of advertising that associates them with outrageous feats, interesting misconceptions have arisen about the products' ingredients and efficacy. The energy drinks in the store refrigerator don't secretly contain banned substances, nor are they made from bull urine—the most common rumor associated with Red Bull. (Red Bull contains a synthetically produced amino acid called taurine. It occurs naturally in the human body, but it was first detected in cattle; hence the name "taurine," as in the constellation of Taurus the Bull, and the urban legend about its source.)

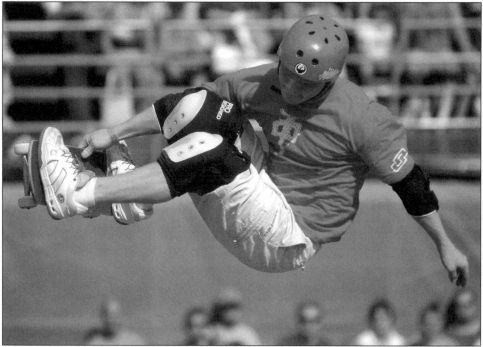

Read the labels and know the ingredients of the energy drinks you use.

Another common misconception in the United States is that this subcategory of energy drink is a new Gen X product. Many energy drinks are new to the U.S. market but have a history of use by athletes in other nations. Dietrick Mateschitz introduced Red Bull to the Austrian market in 1987, and shortly afterward, Red Bull GmbH popularized it throughout Europe. Table 8.1 compares the formulas of energy drinks that feature stimulants and, unlike the carbohydrate and electrolyte drinks covered in earlier chapters, do not focus their product claims on muscle recovery or electrolyte balance.

Products for Young Elite Athletes

Even the young athletes that supplement companies sponsor don't necessarily ingest anything different from the kids on the neighborhood

Table 8.1 Energy Drinks

Product	Energy-related ingredients	Comments/cautions
Battery Energy Drink	Caffeine (135 mg), maltodextrin, sugar, and guarana seed extract	Made in Finland, this drink may not be available everywhere, but it can be ordered via Web sites. With 135 mg of caffeine in an 11.2-oz. serving, in addition to the guarana extract, which is another stimulant, one serving may deliver too much stimulant for small athletes.
BAWLS Guarana Energy	Caffeine, corn syrup, and guarana flavor	Promoted as an adult soft drink that is highly caffeinated.
Hansen's Stamina **Hansen's Energy**	Caffeine, guarana flavor, royal jelly, bee pollen, and L-carnitine Taurine, ginseng, ginkgo biloba, and guarana	These are two of the Hansen's Functionals line, which also includes anti-stress and anti-oxidant drink formulas.
Jones Whoop Ass Energy	Caffeine, high-fructose corn syrup, taurine, royal jelly, guarana extract, ginseng extract, and vitamin B6	None
Red Bull Energy Drink	Caffeine, taurine, and vitamin B6	Claims of improved alertness, reaction time, and stamina are linked to studies.

(continued)

Table 8.1 *(continued)*

Product	Energy-related ingredients	Comments/cautions
Red Devil Energy Drink	Caffeine, taurine, and vitamin B6	None
SoBe Adrenaline Rush Energy Drink	Caffeine, high-fructose corn syrup, taurine, d-ribose, L-carnitine, ginseng, and guarana seed extract	None
Virgin Hi-Energy Drink	Caffeine, taurine, ginseng, and vitamin B6	None
X Drinks	Herbal sources of caffeine and other stimulants (guarana, mate, kava kava, gota kola, betel nut, kola nut, ginseng, ginkgo biloba, green tea)	None

soccer team. For example, E-CAPS sponsors a 12-year-old mountain bike racer from Bozeman, Montana. Before competition and sometimes before training runs, he uses Hammer Gel, an energy gel made by E-CAPS's sister company, Hammer Nutrition. Other than that, his only need for a company product was when he went to the junior nationals in Gainesville, Florida, in August 2001. Faced with the challenge of performing at his best in temperatures that exceeded 100 and humidity over 90 percent, he used an electrolyte replacement drink.

Young Olympians may have a different story, though. In some sports, the biggest difference might be their total caloric intake. The next step up would be a multivitamin, particularly if the athlete's dietary habits or lifestyle are less than ideal. A coach might also introduce supplementation into the program because of deficits induced by unusually heavy training or because they want to see a specific performance-enhancing effect. On the low end, that could be a carbohydrate drink or gel when the athlete is feeling fatigued. On the high end, it could entail a fine-tuned, research-based program, such as the one that swim coach Mike Bottom at the University of California, Berkeley, developed for the U.S. men's Olympic swim team, which brought home gold and silver from Sydney.

Mike awakened to a daunting challenge when he began preparing Gary Hall Jr. and Anthony Ervin—ultimately the joint gold-medal winners of the 50-meter freestyle—and Bart Kizierowski, Gordon Kojulz, and John Olsen for the 2000 summer Olympics:

> When you're an elite athlete, that means you have to compete against the world. As an elite athlete, you are competing against athletes from several countries that are devoting a lot of money, science, time, and energy into developing undetectable or mini-

mally detectable illegal supplements. Right off, you have to know that, and not fool yourself.

You have to be proactive in your pursuit of doing everything legal, and that's not going to harm you, to be a better athlete.

I looked myself in the mirror and said, "As a sprint coach, which is a strength coach—the 50 [meter] freestyle is the strength event in swimming—how am I going to compete against these athletes who are obviously taking growth hormones, Androstenedione, steroids?" Because swimming has such a large aerobic component, even in the sprint, I figured we could compete without doing illegal drugs. But I had to find out for my athletes, what the best route is nutritionally and with supplements, so they could legally and healthfully be the best they could be.

Compounding Mike's challenge was Gary Hall's newly diagnosed case of severe diabetes. Several doctors had told him his swimming career

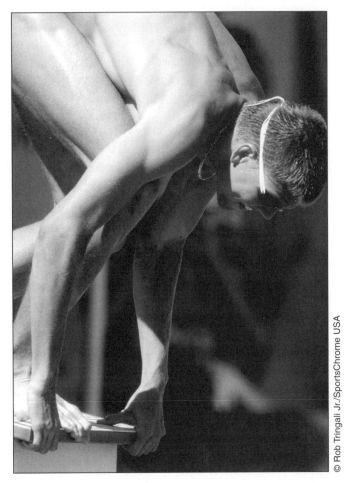

Gary Hall and his coach, Mike Bottom, developed a winning nutrition program to manage his diabetes.

was over, but the nutritional plan that Mike developed helped Gary prove the doctors wrong.

A guiding principle was selecting supplements that would boost the athletes' immune systems, which were taking a beating with the intense training. In other words, recovery products played the central role in the design of the team's sports food program.

After investigating the myriad options available to him, and considering Gary's special health needs, Mike teamed up with four companies: Platinum Performance, New Vision Vitamins, Cytosport, and CellCore.

New Vision Vitamins produced a custom combination of vitamins and minerals for the team. Cytosport provided Cytomax, a carbohydrate/electrolyte drink. Mike was mainly interested in Cytomax's patented method of buffering lactic acid production in the swimmers' muscles. It's meant to reduce the burn during intense training and minimize post-workout soreness. And Platinum Performance and CellCore brought substances that were relatively unknown in the athletic community prior to Mike's use of their products.

Platinum Performance built its line of human supplements after achieving extraordinary success with horses, such as the 2000 Kentucky Derby winner, Fusaichi Pegasus. The company's successful venture into human supplements happened by accident, according to product developer Dr. Doug Herthel, a veterinary surgeon who cofounded the nutrition company with his son, Mark:

> We had a client who was diagnosed with lymphoma. She had a cantaloupe-sized tumor. Part of her work was rehabilitating race-horses after surgery. After 30 years of rehabilitating horses, she saw how well her horses were doing on our nutrition.
>
> When she was diagnosed and first started chemotherapy, she was having a terrible time. Unbeknownst to me, she started eating the horse product. She's a very sharp horse person—she saw what it did for her horses and wanted the same benefits. I noticed that she was doing very well, but didn't talk too much about it. One day, at the end of her chemotherapy, she came to me and said, "You won't believe this, but I haven't lost a day of work. All through my chemo, I've been active; I've been to Europe, Hong Kong, and the East Coast selling horses. All through my illness, I've been eating your horse product." That's when I decided to make it for people.

The Platinum sports food that the swim team adopted was based on a product called Granular. Granular was originally developed to enhance bone and tissue healing in horses, although it's had the corollary benefit of extending the performance life of horses. Because Doug's practice centered on care for prize-winning sport horses, some worth millions of dollars, his product research and design reflected the lofty expectations of their owners. He formulated Granular to supply all the essential oils, vitamins, amino acids, and fiber, as well as the trace minerals, antioxidants, and joint-protecting factors. Sick and injured horses who received it at the clinic rebounded from treatment faster, healing quicker and with fewer complications. That meant they returned to work faster—actually showing more muscle growth and higher performance than before they entered the clinic—to earn their keep through racing, jumping, competing in endurance events, or doing whatever each one did best. In the case of Fusaichi Pegasus, Doug performed surgery in the summer of 1999 to take care of bone chips and synovitis in the horse's ankle. By the end of the summer, supported by the Granular product, Fusaichi Pegasus returned to training. By year's end, he returned to competition. The following May, he won the Derby.

Doug's design philosophy for this and other Platinum products is "Everything works in synergy, and the cells need everything. A product is incomplete if it omits one or two key items." From a commercial perspective, there's a downside to including "everything" and not using chemical preservatives to lock in the integrity of the ingredients: The product does not have the shelf life of many other products that are considered meal replacements. It's made to order and shipped immediately; it isn't meant to sit around.

The Platinum bar that the swim team chose has the same components as Granular, but they're more concentrated. It would be classified as a meal replacement, but (as of this writing) its formula differs markedly from other meal replacement bars on the market, because it includes omega-3 bioactive essential lipids. While that ingredient greatly elevates the bar's nutritional value, it also makes it more vulnerable to spoiling. Natural preservatives such as tumeric and pine bark help the ingredients retain their integrity for four months, but the bar isn't sold in stores, where shelf life is measured in a year or more. On the other hand, the bar is far from delicate. Cassandra Lowe, the Australian cyclist, packed the bars on her bike as she rode in the 2000 Race Across America. She ate a bar about once every two hours as she peddled to victory in 10 days and three hours.

The macronutrient profile of this bar also separates it from others and makes it well suited for endurance athletes of any age who engage in extremely intense training and competitive events. A 25-gram bar—less than half the size of most bars—offers 90 calories, half of which are from fat. Of that total, 27 calories (three grams) come from healthful omega-3 lipids; on the other end of the spectrum, fewer than five calories (one-half gram) come from saturated fat. A serious athlete should keep saturated fats to a minimum; among other reasons, they slow nutrient absorption. The bar also provides four grams of protein, four grams of fiber, and six grams of carbohydrates.

Platinum produced an HMB compound called Myo-Fuel to promote the athletes' recovery. Myo-Fuel contains glutamine to help build muscles, plus the antioxidant vitamins E and C. Doug points out that HMB, which is nearly a staple among strength athletes, was originally developed by a veterinarian to improve muscle in livestock so that they would yield more meat.

The team also took Platinum's Hemo-Flo to help their bodies produce nitric oxide and to support optimal blood flow. These capsules feature a combination of amino acids and antioxidants that qualify it as a medical food of the same ilk as CookePharma's HeartBar, a product designed for patients with angina and other circulation disorders. A main ingredient is L-arginine, the amino acid that stimulates production of nitric oxide, which is a major vasodilator (that is, something that expands the blood vessels in the body) (Furchgott et al. 1998). By allowing the cells to produce more nitric acid, it relaxes muscle constriction; that's why people with angina or peripheral artery disease—or diabetics like Gary Hall—benefit from it. The Hemo-Flo also contains L-glutamine, vitamins C and E, tumeric, uncaria, and pine bark. Tumeric and pine bark, as mentioned above, are natural preservatives with nutritional value. Tumeric is the spice that gives curry powder its dark yellow color, and it is used in many herbal anti-inflammatory formulas. Studies have shown that it can hold its own in comparisons with prescription nonsteroidal anti-inflammatory drugs; unlike many NSAIDs, it doesn't lead to stomach upset. Uncaria is more commonly known as Cat's Claw, an herb that's native to South and Central America and recognized for its ability to strengthen the immune system. Pine bark extract, taken from the maritime pine tree, is an antioxidant. (Further discussion of such substances can be found in chapter 10.)

Cellcore USA was the final corporate partner Mike chose for the team. Cellcore's product, which is better known in Japan than in North America or Europe, is water. Specifically, the product is micro-clustered water, developed by a process for which inventor Dr. Lee H. Lorenzen received a United States Patent on January 27, 1998. With his micro-clustered water, Lee aims to address the problem of dehydration on a cellular level. His goal is to restructure water so that it passes into the cells more effectively. For athletes, the important thing to know is that most people past childhood—even those who regularly drink water—are somewhat dehydrated, and that condition impedes athletic performance and undermines overall health.

By including CellCore's micro-clustered water in his team's nutrition regimen, Mike tried to enhance two physiological processes for the swimmers—both byproducts of keeping them hydrated at the cellular level. Their intense training created a lactate environment, and the challenge was to maintain good muscle performance even in an almost anaerobic state. In the 50-meter freestyle, they wouldn't have time to make up an oxygen debt in the seconds that they would be swimming; they would have to be able to keep their muscles functioning. They would also have to realize a full recovery afterward. By drinking micro-clustered water, they hoped to absorb nutrients more effectively so that vitamins and minerals would work better. They also wanted to trigger a cell-dumping effect. After a race or training session, cells would eliminate waste more rapidly and new fluids would flush back in, thus improving recovery time.

Lee emphasizes that these effects can be documented: "We can measure the impedance of the muscle tissue and look at the electrolyte balance and show very substantial changes in the ratios within a few minutes."

A biochemist by training, Lee's drive to develop the water was fueled by frustration and intellectual curiosity, not by a desire to sell water to athletes:

> The motivation for developing the micro-clustered water was my wife. Regardless of what we tried, she continued to spiral downward with chronic fatigue and fibromyalgia. Dehydration is a very serious problem for people with these illnesses, but if you rehydrate them too quickly, they will actually get worse. You can't merely flush water through the outer cell space. You have to transport it in. I was frustrated that we couldn't find anything to help her.

In the mid-1980s, when his wife's degeneration and pain became serious, Lee worked as a researcher in pharmacology, helping to develop new medications. He says he was very "hard headed" about using the knowledge associated with his profession to try to help her, and "she suffered through several years because of that." They even began exhausting therapies outside of Western mainstream medicine, such as acupuncture and homeopathy.

> As a last resort, I was going to take her to France to the healing springs of Lourdes. Before we did that, I called a geophysicist friend of mine. We had searched out all the healing springs of the world that were known at that time. I asked him to do a geological survey to find out if there were any similarities to the geology that might explain the emergence of these springs in these particular locations. He found, first of all, that the sources of all these waters were very, very deep, under very high pressure, bubbling up through magnetizing quartz, and they're cold. The other interesting thing is that

the healing effects of the solutions only last minutes. If you drink from the source, you can benefit, but if you try to take it with you, it doesn't work. This is why scientists have dismissed waters as only having a placebo effect. If something is changing within minutes, it can't be mineral or bacterial or any common factor like that. It had to be something in the water itself. That's when we started looking at the clustering effect, and indeed, that's what we found.

Another peculiarity that visitors to healing springs like Lourdes have experienced is that the water evaporates like alcohol off their skin. This is because the clusters in the water are so small, that the water has a lower surface tension than other water.

In trying to duplicate what nature had done, as well as stabilize it, Lee had a team of scientists collect healing waters from all over the world. At a facility, they used a method that Lee developed with a biophysicist from Japan to extract the water from the source so that it would not lose its integrity. Essentially, within a fraction of a second of drawing the water, they would flash freeze it with liquid nitrogen. They could then transport it back to Lee's lab to examine the crystalline structures of the water and photograph them using an electron microscope.

The greatest payoff for Lee is that his wife has shown almost no symptoms of the diseases since she began drinking just two glasses of the water a day. "She's not cured, but she has energy and feels good. But when she stops drinking the solution, within a few days, she feels run down and pain returns."

In terms of athletes, the prime candidates for Lee's solutions are competitors in sports that involve a sudden buildup of lactic acid. If you are in a sport where you have to go into the anaerobic energy zone, you may want to try this product. The cost per bottle is about three times the cost of commercially bottled spring water, but you don't have to drink much of it on a daily basis to get the benefits.

Young children, like fruit on the tree and vegetables just after harvesting, have this kind of small-clustered water present in them. After the age of 35, however, the content drops precipitously. Blood becomes more sluggish, slowing down a lot of body functions. One way to help counter the effects is through aerobic exercise, which Lee says "helps to mobilize water in an efficient way." It doesn't solve the age-related problem, but it definitely helps.

The chart on page 169 summarizes the program that swimming coach Mike Bottom used to support the U.S. Olympic team's successful performance in the Sydney Olympics.

The 2000 Olympics U.S. Men's Swim Team Supplement Program

Multivitamin/mineral: New Vision Vitamins
Nutrient-dense sports foods: Platinum Performance Granular and Bars
Muscle recovery and development supplement: Platinum Performance Myo-Fuel
Circulation supplement: Platinum Performance Hemo-Flo
Carbohydrate/electrolyte drink: Cytosport's Cytomax
Water: Cellcore's Vivo Ready-to-Drink

Courtesy of Mike Bottom, University of California, Berkeley, California.

A Supplement to Avoid

Young athletes need to know what to avoid as much as what will enhance performance. If you are still in your teens, don't even consider doing pro-hormones. They are completely wrong for you and could actually undermine your optimal development. If you are in your early 20s and are thinking about using them, talk to a physician and your coach. It's possible that the substances won't do you any good, or that you will violate the first principle of sports foods: Do no harm. Plenty of products are better matched to your needs and level of physical development to help you make the jump from dreams to medals.

As Mike Bottom points out, you have to have your head in the sand not to recognize that people who do banned anabolic substances show up at elite events like the Olympics. There are many ways to beat drug tests, and some countries covertly invest lots of money in perfecting them. But when Mike put his athletes in the pool in Sydney, they proved that they could achieve gold-medal performance on legal and healthful supplements.

Peak Performance in the Masters Years

The higher the age of an athlete, regardless of fitness levels, the lower the level of certain substances in the body that contribute to peak performance. Combine that fact with the desire of many elite athletes in their 30s, 40s, and beyond to maintain an extremely high level of fitness, and you design a major nutritional challenge. Athletes past their 20s face lifestyle and workout issues as well. You can't get away with slipping into some of the bad habits that younger athletes do, nor can you routinely recover from high-stress workouts as you might have done earlier in your athletic career.

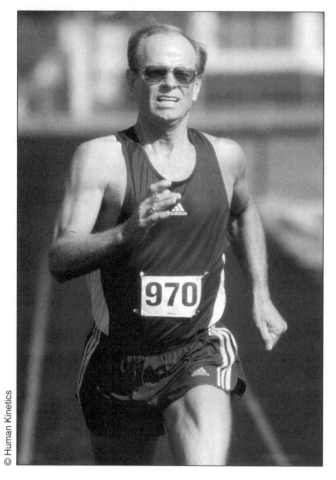

© Human Kinetics

Nutritional supplements can provide a tool to offset some of the disadvantages of aging.

But there is plenty of good news. Nate Llerandi, a successful triathlon coach, observes:

> There are degenerative issues that happen as we age, but training and proper diet will stem the tide of that, or at least slow it down. I now see athletes in their late 30s and early 40s who are doing things that, 10 years ago [in the early 1990s], nobody would have expected from somebody of that age. I think we have learned to help counter degeneration processes.

The proof is everywhere, including in some of the world's toughest races, such as the Badwater/Whitney 135, the brutal desert race that loses top competitors to stomach distress, dehydration, vertigo, stress fractures, and foot disorders, to name just a few likely race-enders. In the 1999 Hi-Tec Badwater/Whitney event, 6 of the top 10 finishers were over 40 at race time, and three were over 50. The top man was 41 and the top woman—the remarkable endurance athlete, Angelika Casteneda, who set another record—was 56.

The Furnace Creek 508 (miles) is the cycling counterpart to Badwater, both of which force athletes to endure the heat of Death Valley and the altitude of the mountains. Nate Llerandi coached the 1999 course record holder, Jim "Pterodactyl" Petri. Jim, who is in his 60s, says his nutritional keys to success were taking in 500 calories an hour, drinking lots of water, taking E-CAPS supplements, and drinking Coca-Cola when he felt drowsy.

One of the first companies in the industry, E-CAPS has developed a following with masters athletes, even though its products are designed for endurance athletes of all ages. Part of the reason is undoubtedly the company's association with high-profile nutritionist and masters athlete, Dr. Bill Misner. (Bill, who was born in 1939, backs up his academic and sports-medicine training credentials with masters running and cycling championships.) A more fundamental reason is that cofounder Brian Frank has considered the biomarkers of aging in developing his product line. His products increase the efficiency with which an athlete's body operates, so that it can handle greater workloads, recover from them more quickly, and maintain a high degree of overall health.

Brian began exploring the potential benefits of nutritional supplements in the 1980s, principally to try to create competitive advantages for himself in his endurance sports. He and his father introduced their first product, Race Caps, in August of 1987 at the Coors Classic, an event where Brian and Jennifer (Biddulph) Maxwell also tried to bring their "powerful bars" to the attention of the racing world. At the time, classically trained nutritionists like Jennifer were very skeptical about the value of the Franks' supplements. They thought that a balanced diet should provide all the nutrients that a healthy athlete would require. In contrast, Brian and his father, a successful chiropractor, believed that intense training creates the need for supplementation, no matter how well you eat—just as athletes and sports nutrition experts believe today.

"We saw too many athletes who were teetering on that fine line between peak fitness and being sick from overtraining," Brian recalls. Unfortunately, the options for an endurance athlete in 1987 were slim. Bodybuilders had protein powder, but until the arrival of PowerBar, endurance athletes only had products like Gatorade and Exceed to meet their special energy and nutrient requirements. Brian explains,

> There was nothing in the way of supplements that would address the unique needs of endurance athletes. We felt those needs were very different from those of strength athletes because of the volume they train, the type of free radicals their activities are creating, and so forth. So we set out to develop phase-effective, ergogenic aids that would be specifically geared toward the needs and requirements of endurance athletes.

Within a year of when we got started, there was the Ben Johnson steroid scandal at the Seoul Olympics, so there was a lot of focus on drugs. I can't tell you how many times people would walk by our table at an event and say, "Oh, yeah, that stuff's probably just a bunch of steroids." In some ways, maybe that scandal was good for all of us in that athletes became more aware of supplements and ergogenic aids—both illicit and legal.

Snapshots of Super Master's Diets

Bill Misner's own diet is a good basis for understanding how a masters endurance athlete might combine whole foods with supplements that mitigate the effects of aging. Admittedly, his diet would represent an extreme for most people, but consider carefully how it addresses both the health and performance issues of a 60-plus male who runs about 50 miles a week in addition to strength and speed workouts.

In planning his diet, as well as in advising other athletes, Bill thinks in terms of Optimum Daily Allowances (ODAs). In the context of ODAs, the ideal amount of nutrients depends on considerations that include age, activity, performance goals, and medical conditions. In addition, the ODAs don't portray fat as merely saturated or unsaturated, as the RDAs do. You learn very little about designing a high-performance diet from an RDA that simply says that, for a 2,000-calorie diet, your total fat intake should be about 66 grams, with your saturated fat intake not exceeding 22 grams. In contrast, an ODA discussion of fat offers specifics in terms of omega-3, omega-6, trans-fatty acid, and more. The ODAs for omega-3 and omega-6 start at about five grams and two grams, respectively, and for trans-fatty acid, they start at zero grams. Trans-fatty acids trick the body into using them in building cell membranes, which then have a reduced ability to allow trace minerals to penetrate. Results could be cell death or a diseased state—important outcomes to avoid, particularly if you are attempting to stave off the degenerative effects of aging to stay competitive. Trans-fatty acids are formed when liquid fats, such as vegetable oils, are hardened by hydrogenation to produce margarine and other products.

Bill's own diet clearly reflects this concept of totally avoiding bad nutrients and consuming megadoses of some good nutrients, as shown on page 173.

On an occasional basis, Bill will take 2,400 milligrams of arginine–pyroglutamate-lysine (APGL). This measure is another age-related choice. Substantial research, some of which was done in the early 1980s, has looked at how taking such amino acid combinations orally stimulates the

Bill Misner's Average Training Day Diet

Morning

2–3 pieces of fruit at various times

Noon

6- to 12-mile run

Post-workout

Bob's Red Mill 5-grain cereal (organic triticale, quinoa, oats, flax, and rolled barley), into which Bill mixes almonds, pumpkin seeds, sunflower seeds, and a combination of soy and whey protein (25 gm each). He sweetens the mixture with Hammer Gel to create a very small insulin spike, which drives the carbohydrates as they digest over the next two hours back into the glycogen supply to help with the following day's workout.

Multivitamin/mineral

Bill takes E-CAPS Premium Insurance Caps, which are formulated using the ODA, not the RDA. An example of the difference is that two packets (one serving) of the E-CAPS multi provides 1,000 mg of vitamin C in the form of calcium ascorbate and 1,000 mg of bioflavonoids, whereas the RDAs call for just 60 mg. The product also has chelated minerals and boron. Chelation is the process of bonding a mineral to an amino acid to make it easier to digest and assimilate. "Boron is a necessary substrate for anabolic hormones as well as a number of other hormone mechanisms," explains Bill, who advises a dosage of 3–5 mg daily. "This is especially important for women. It is more a factor in the female hormone mechanisms than male."

2 gm of essential fatty acids

Coenzyme Q10

Co Q10 levels drop with age; the supplement should be taken with fat to metabolize it properly.

1 Enduro Cap

The key ingredient in E-CAPS Enduro Caps is Cytochrome C, a coenzyme found in the highest concentrations in the muscles and a key component in the respiratory chain. It is responsible for recycling ATP in the muscle and, along with Coenzyme Q10, initiates the transfer of your body's main fuel source within the working muscles.

5 mg of piperine

Also known as biopherine, this substance is a component of black pepper. Studies have shown piperine increases the absorption rate of nutrients.

2 capsules of "good bacteria"

Bill takes E-CAPS' Digest Caps, which contains L. Acidophilus, B. Bifidum, and B. Longum. For an endurance athlete, such a product promotes efficient digestion and assimilation of nutrients during both training and competition. A balance of good bacterial microorganisms aids digestion, cholesterol levels, immune system response, and vitamin and mineral absorption rates.

(continued)

(continued)

A digestive enzyme

Bill emphasizes that this choice reflects his 60+ age. He says a younger athlete probably wouldn't need it.

1 capsule of rosemary extract

The carnoseic acid in rosemary is thought by some people, including Bill, to be an anti-aging product. He wants to keep it in his system continually because it is "related to a number of blood factors."

1 capsule tumeric extract

Some of the benefits of tumeric were referenced in the discussion of the Platinum products used by the U.S. Men's Swim Team, but Bill's reason for including it is a little different. His interest in the herb is that a small amount of tumeric each day is supposed to keep levels of the blood-clotting agent fibrinogen in check. High levels of fibrinogen predispose you to coronary and cerebral artery disease.

4 grams of vitamin C

400 IU of vitamin E

1 gram of fat-soluble, powdered vitamin C

Evening (3 hours before bedtime)

Same supplements as post-workout, noontime meal

Liquid, sublingual vitamin B-12

This is important because Bill, the son of a butcher, almost never eats red meat.

A vegetable/fruit medley, such as organic peas, corn, broccoli, carrots, one tomato (every night), and olives for omega-9

Kidney or black beans, or albacore tuna

Courtesy of Bill Misner, E-Caps Inc. & Hammer Nutrition LTD., Whitefish, Montana.

body's secretion of human growth hormone (HGH). As athletes age, any healthful way to promote HGH production will give them an edge. Alternatively, Bill sometimes takes 2,000 milligrams of glutamine to boost his growth hormone release. These supplements must be taken on an empty stomach to be effective, because growth hormone and insulin "don't get along," as Bill points out.

> For an old guy like me, it's a safe way to get [HGH] into the system. It's especially important if I'm doing a strength workout or a speed workout, or if it's just the middle of the week and I need to boost the cumulative effects prior to my long run on the weekends.

> I think growth hormone is a big part of a strength or speed session because, as an endurance athlete, you're looking at these sessions to improve your pace.

At bedtime, Bill also takes 10 milligrams of melatonin, which he feels provides a growth hormone advantage. As he's gotten older, he has had a harder time sleeping through an entire night. He feels that if he gets a deeper sleep at night, then the growth hormone is released at a higher rate. ZMA is another possible choice for the same reason, but Bill doesn't use it because of a personal test that he conducted, which involved himself and another masters endurance champion. Their experience was that their testosterone levels actually went down with ZMA use, in sharp contrast to the young football players who participated in the original study that validated claims of its anabolic benefits. Reasons for the difference could be twofold:

1. Bill and his fellow masters champion are older men, with different hormone mechanisms from the young athletes.
2. The endurance sports they do expend a high amount of calories but require relatively little growth hormone.

Regardless of this possible effect, endurance athletes of all ages and both genders need to pay attention to their zinc and chromium levels, both of which are depleted through intense training.

Bill's attention to HGH reflects a harsh reality for any male athlete over the age of 25. Testosterone levels peak in the male body in the late teens and early 20s and then steadily decline. The stress of intense training tends to further depress hormone levels. Male strength and endurance athletes in their mid-30s and above who don't have a training and nutrition program consistent with their needs commonly find that their usual 8 to 10 hours a week of intense training robs them of a libido. If your testosterone level is so low that you have no sexual desire, think of the consequences on your body's ability to build and maintain muscle and do all the other functions that testosterone is a critical part of. Diminished workload capacity, an inability to recover from stress—these are just some of reasons that have sent men over 30 in search of anabolic steroids and prohormones. As Bill points out, however, they are not the only options.

Female masters athletes have another key age-related consideration. To avert stress fractures, female runners must complement their endurance training with weight-bearing exercises when they hit their mid-30s. Even supported by a diet that includes calcium supplementation, a running program is not enough to force the body to retain bone integrity. Decreasing hormone levels as menopause approaches can also affect a female athlete's ability to compete effectively as a strength or endurance athlete.

It is interesting to see the remarkable similarities, as well as the differences, between Bill's daily food and supplement program and that of Dr. Paul Hutinger, a top masters swimmer who, as of this writing, is 76 years old. Paul taught exercise physiology at Western Illinois University before retiring. Before a meet or training session, he might have a piece of whole-grain toast, a banana, and a cup of coffee. Immediately after his workout, he takes in some carbs and protein to boost recovery, often in the form of a Clif Bar. When he gets home, he eats oatmeal and fruit, and later, a simple dinner that follows a 40-30-30 macronutrient distribution.

The big difference between Paul's supplementation program and Bill's is the inclusion of saw palmetto, which Paul began taking in his 60s to mitigate prostate problems. Even though he has dabbled in DHEA use—he found that it didn't make any difference—and does use glutamine regularly to aid recovery, he somehow escaped the sharp decline in testosterone levels that most men experience. When Paul was in his 60s, he participated in studies on testosterone levels conducted at Western Illinois University and found he was "in the 900 range—like a teenager." (The normal range for a 30-year-old man is 250 to 400.) Nevertheless, Paul suggests that many older male and female athletes might benefit from carefully regulated DHEA use.

Young, Old, and in Between

Age is among the key considerations in determining what sports foods can make a profound difference in your performance. Clearly, young athletes face the lowest level of complexity in terms of diet and supplementation, with competitive preteens needing nothing but a good diet and the occasional electrolyte replacement, multivitamin, and energy bar or gel. But as athletes hit the 20s and take on more intense competition, the secrets of world-class athletes can help them get an edge: Even at that early age, certain body systems are starting to degenerate and can benefit from the right performance-enhancing foods. The biomarkers of aging point to the need for more antioxidants, immune system boosters, and joint protection for athletes in their 40s, and nutrition can get really complicated by the time an elite athlete enters masters competitions.

Regardless of your age, the key to getting good results from supplements is using them consistently. During the season or phase of your life that you commit to a supplement program, make it an integral part of your schedule.

CHAPTER 9

Refueling During Competition

Non-endurance competitions generally involve stops and starts for athletes—innings, shifts from offense to defense, or player substitutions. Even some endurance sports involve downtime. In a multi-day adventure race, for example, you might encounter a mandatory stop until daylight because your team has reached the whitewater section of the racecourse. All of these inactivity periods give you some flexibility in refueling; convenient packaging may not be a dominant issue. On the other hand, marathoners go nonstop, and tennis players go nonstop until a set is over. They have to grab something quickly and move on, so choices are limited. Many extreme sports last less than a minute, so refueling during competition is not an issue—unless you look at competition as encompassing the hours of heats, or preliminary runs, in which you have to stay sharp to stay in the games. In some way, that challenge is similar to that of a power lifter or bodybuilder. For all of these athletes, starts must be quick and downtimes can last more than an hour.

The following considerations shape the discussion of refueling during competition:

• Athletes in 90-minute to three-hour games with timeouts don't necessarily need or want solid food. Water or a carbohydrate drink supplemented with electrolytes should often be sufficient; the electrolyte replacement becomes more important if you're playing in the heat. But should the drink have protein as well as carbs? Will herbs help give you a boost on the field?

• Endurance athletes and players who go nonstop for the same period of time face glycogen depletion as well as the loss of fluid and electrolytes, so a carbohydrate/electrolyte drink makes a lot of sense.

During competition, however, the concentration of carbs in the drink can make the big difference between refueling efficiently and slowing down or cramping. Here again, you face the question of herbs or no herbs.

• Competitors in a multi-day footrace, like the Marathon de Sables, or a multisport, 10- or 12-day adventure race, like the Eco-Challenge or Elf Authentic Adventure, want solid food in addition to liquids. It really is not just a matter of need; it's a matter of want. I know because I tried to live on a liquid sports food during the first few days of Eco-Challenge in southern Utah; I was ready to eat rocks just to give my jaws exercise. With all those days of nearly nonstop activity, what is the best solid food to bring along? Do specially formulated products make sense as the sole food source?

• In terms of training, power lifters may share a lot with football players, but during competition, the demand is one big anaerobic moment in each phase of the competition. Nutritionally, you need to support maximum effort for a handful of seconds. The trick is, you don't really know how long you will have between lifts.

• The timing issue affects many extreme sports competitors, as well—skateboarders, sky surfers, stunt bikers, and so on—who might go all out in a 50-second heat but then have to sit around for an hour or two before the next round. Even though the timing challenge may be similar to that of power lifters, the energy challenge is different. With stunt-oriented events, you're working intensely but probably more in the aerobic zone, and the requirements for balance and timing mean that control is critical.

• Finally, there are the bodybuilders. If you've never competed as a bodybuilder, spending the morning running through compulsory positions and the evening presenting a flexing routine to music, you have no idea how taxing it is. You stand under hot lights holding different poses, which are powerful isometric actions. I've seen little pools of sweat form at the feet of these athletes. After a round, you walk off and wait and wait until it's your turn again. That process goes on for the good part of a day, during which your thoughts are a web of superstitions and honest fears, such as, "If I drink water, my cuts won't be as sharp. If I eat a banana now, I might have to go to the bathroom when I'm on stage."

Refueling Opportunities

By categorizing sports in terms of refueling opportunities, table 9.1 is meant to help you organize your thinking about matching performance-enhancing products to your competitive situation. Although this is not a comprehensive list of sports—nor does it necessarily reflect how intensely you personally play a particular sport—the table suggests that there are six different ways to look at your chances to refuel during an activity:

1. Periodic/constant. Slow periods of activity or periodic breaks in play allow maximum flexibility in terms of when and what you eat. Many sports can be enjoyed this way; the ones listed in the table represent several that allow casual participants or moderately competitive athletes plenty of time to refuel. Of course, at the professional level these sports would fall into other categories. For example, even though sailing made the list, if you're racing in the America's Cup, you clearly don't have the same opportunities to eat as someone out for a casual afternoon on calm water.

2. Periodic/occasional. Sports that periodically rely on the anaerobic energy systems dominate this category. The one-repetition, maximum lift in a strength contest; the allout rush to tackle a running back with the football; the 50-meter sprint across the pool—these efforts are in the context of competitions with some downtime but moments of great intensity.

3. Periodic/constrained. In this category, you find activities that involve extreme environments or athletic apparatus that limits the opportunity to eat or drink.

4. Nearly continuous/constant. Generally speaking, you can set an individual pace and degree of difficulty in these sports. The exertion is nearly continuous, but there are no rules about minutes of play, nor are there necessarily environmental conditions that inhibit your ability to eat or drink.

5. Nearly continuous/occasional. In terms of duration, this category includes two different types of activities. The first type is endurance events that offer extended periods of time when refueling is theoretically possible, even though you may continue to race while you're eating. Whether or not you take advantage of the opportunities to refuel depends on how hard you're pushing to win or get to the next checkpoint. The other type is competitions that last more than an hour and that involve almost constant movement until the end of the quarter, the game, or whatever period of play applies.

6. Nearly continuous/constrained. In this case, the constraint does not hinge on environmental or gear-related factors as much as on the nature of the sport itself. You are constantly on the move; you don't have time to think about eating, much less do it.

Table 9.1   Refueling Opportunities

	Constant	Occasional	Constrained
Periodic exertion	Bowling	Football	High-altitude mountaineering
	Golf	Power lifting	Whitewater kayaking
	Cross-country skiing	Gymnastics	Whitewater rafting
	Sailing	Skateboarding	Hang gliding
	Expedition kayaking	Rollerblading	Paragliding
		Wrestling	Scuba diving
		Baseball	
		Cricket	
		Bodybuilding	
		Olympic lifting	
		Fencing	
		Sprints (swimming, running, cycling, skating)	
Nearly continuous exertion	Rock climbing	Adventure racing	Swimming
	Cycling	Sled-dog racing	Auto racing
	Marathon	Triathlon	Boxing
		Ultramarathon	Aerobatic flying
		Basketball	Surfing
		Tennis	Downhill skiing
		Soccer	Snowboarding
		Polo	Downhill mountain biking
		Rugby	
		Handball	

Competition Fueling: Advice for Everyone

Don't introduce new products or patterns of eating or drinking during a competition. You might get sick or weaken yourself to the point where you lose energy and your performance drops. The key is to get your body acclimated to certain products so that you can predictably boost your energy when you need to. Part of your competitive edge includes finding out who the race or event sponsors are, so that you know what to expect during the game or along the racecourse. If Gatorade is the sponsor, for example, get used to it in advance. If it's a new product, try to get samples, or train with something as close to the formula as you can. To some extent, you can train your body to use and want certain products.

One year at the Hawaii Ironman, MET-Rx came in as a sponsor and offered its new ORS (Oral Rehydration System) drink along the course. The athletes didn't have previous access to the drink, which is a significant reason why a number of them became ill. Tony DeBoom found he was reacting badly to it, so he switched to the available alternative—water. He still felt strong coming off the bike leg, holding a solid fourth place. The run, however, became a torture test. Drinking only water had flushed his system to the point where he suffered from hyponeutremia,

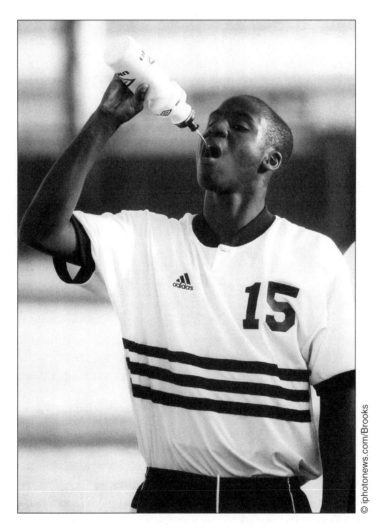

© iphotonews.com/Brooks

"Hydration" means more than drinking just water if your exercise is protracted, intense, or in extreme temperatures.

a potentially a life-threatening condition caused by a serious loss of sodium. Heaving, feeling bloated, and completely fatigued, he collapsed on the side of the road.

This experience leads to another guideline for all athletes: Proper hydration is the foundation of any high-performance nutrition program. Whether you're a tennis player, a power lifter, or a bodybuilder, liquids are your friends during competition as much as they are during training. Caffeine and creatine increase the amount of water you need to keep your energy high, so you will need to adjust accordingly. Two major signs point to lack of sufficient hydration: fatigue and yellow urine. Very dark urine is a symptom of a potentially fatal lack of fluids called rhabdomyolysis. Constipation is a big hint, too.

Periodic Exertion/Constant Refueling Opportunities

Some sports are paced in such a way that casual athletes usually associate them with eating and drinking. In fact, many people see bowling, golf, and sailing primarily as good excuses to have a few beers with friends. The issue is a little more complicated for serious athletes—instead of beer, the drink of choice should be water. On a brutally hot day on the golf course or on the boat, you might also want to take a sports drink that will help replenish your electrolytes.

Periodic Exertion/Occasional Refueling Opportunities

In an explosive-action sport, you may be tempted to refuel with a product that delivers an energy spike, something that jacks up the adrenaline. Sack that quarterback! Nail that deadlift! Your inclination might be to use products in liquid or capsule form that feature ma huang and guarana seed extracts, for example, both of which are powerful herbal stimulants. Go down this path cautiously: Make sure you use them in training first or you might face performance problems during the competition. Don't use them at all if the NCAA sanctions your competition or if your goal is Olympic lifting. The IOC considers ma huang an illegal substance.

First, consider the health risks exacerbated by competition. In a sport that requires a one-repetition maximum or the rough equivalent (for example, an allout push to down the ball carrier), you are driving your heart as hard as it will go. In the heat of competition, you might extend yourself well beyond anything you've done in practice. Add to that the extra adrenaline you're pumping because this is "the real thing" rather than practice, and your body may not be able to handle the same amount or type of stimulant you use in training.

For some of the same reasons, you could actually lose a competitive edge by using the product, or by using too much of it. You need to feel powerful for a single moment in time, not hyperactive, like the human equivalent of a beehive that's been poked with a broomstick. There's a mental aspect to this, too, that is very important. I know from personal experience in power lifting that a big part of success in the lift is the ability to focus the mind—to visualize the weight moving and direct mental power to the muscles. If you are jittery from your sports drink or capsule, that feeling could ruin your concentration.

Because you will have to deliver explosive bursts of energy—you will be working in the anaerobic zone during part of your competition—think about what you can do before the day of the event to help you. As indicated in earlier chapters, some top athletes use creatine supplementation (or perhaps creatine loading) in the weeks before the competition. They believe that, at the moment they need an explosion of energy, the added creatine helps them pull through.

Drink water during your breaks, regardless of the ambient temperature, but stay away from anything that could bloat you, like a carbonated beverage. If you get hungry or feel your energy fading, eat light. Try a sports gel with your water. The 100 calories will cut your hunger a little and give you an energy boost. During a competition, even if you are only competing for short periods throughout the day, you are better off hungry than having your body expend the effort it takes to digest a meal.

Swimmer Dara Torres took a somewhat unusual approach to fueling before her events in the Sydney Olympics, where she won gold in the 4 × 100 meter freestyle and individual medley relays and individual bronzes in the 100 meter butterfly, 100 meter freestyle, and 50 meter freestyle. Equipped with a newly developed formula from GU called Hard Rock, which contains more amino acids than the standard GU, she relied on an energy-gel loading program:

> I'd take one packet an hour and a half before I'd swim in a race, one packet 45 minutes before, and one packet 10 to 15 minutes before. I'd also take one immediately after for recovery.

Seek out gels without simple sugars if you want to try a program like this. Also keep in mind that Bill Vaughan at GU actually developed the Hard Rock product with elite athletes in mind; it differs in several ways from commercially available GU.

There are also tips that you don't want to try. Some athletes—football players, in particular—have superstitiously turned to pickle juice as a substitute for water or an electrolyte replacement drink. Pickle juice became a "secret weapon" after the Philadelphia Eagles admitted swigging it during a game in October 2000, when they brought down the Dallas Cowboys. Each two-ounce shot, roughly the size they drank, contains about 700 milligrams of sodium, which is about the same amount that 1.5 liters of Gatorade provides. If you're a well-hydrated player approaching 300 pounds, then maybe you could try the pickle juice—after you talk to your coach. If you don't meet that description, stay with water. Too much sodium in your system can cause problems. An excess of sodium will upset your electrolyte balance by drawing water and potassium out of your cells. Another effect, which you may have experienced after eating salty food, is that too much sodium will cause water to collect in and around your body tissues, and you'll feel sluggish.

Periodic Exertion/Constrained Refueling Opportunities

In this context, "constrained" means that you are in an environment like raging rapids or using some apparatus like a hang glider that seriously limits your options on refueling, even though your level of exertion may not. If your sport fits in this category, your nutritional considerations are rather basic: what you can eat to make sure your brain has the sugar it needs to function, and how you can effectively hydrate. After that, depending on the duration of the adventure, your concern is to prevent muscle wasting, or catabolism.

When Will Gadd paraglides into the record books, as he has several times, he is airborne for hours at a time. He also spends a lot of that time at altitudes where the temperature is at or below freezing, even though it may be 100 degrees on the ground. His drinks of choice are Red Bull and water, and his snacks can be anything, as long as they stay soft and are easy to handle: "I scattered a lot of M&Ms over a field one day. M&Ms don't work. It's hard to chew them because your face is cold."

Mountaineers face a more extreme version of this dilemma when they reach altitudes on Everest and K2 where energy bars are among the many food items that become inedible. When you venture into frigid temperatures, foods that can serve you well are energy gels, which might become more viscous but won't freeze solid, and sweetened condensed milk. Several gel manufacturers now produce squeezable containers with straws or hoses so that you don't have to rely on tiny packets when you're on the side of a big mountain.

Nearly Continuous Exertion/Constant Refueling Opportunities

Describing refueling opportunities as "constant" for any sport that involves almost continuous exertion is more of a technicality than a reality. In a marathon or cycling race, for example, you do the best you can at points along the course to ingest nutrition—and you must do it. In

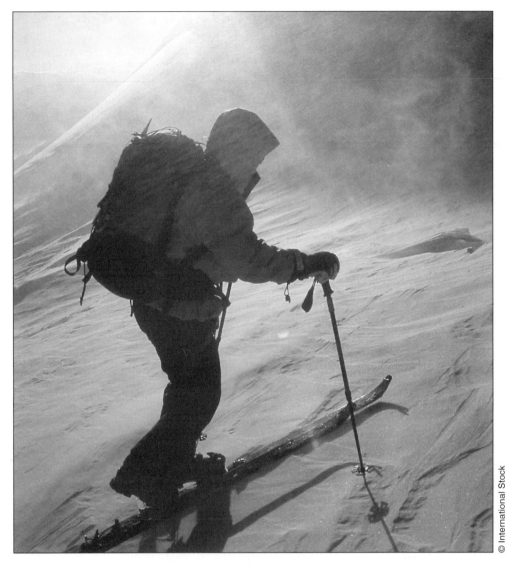

© International Stock

Remember to stay hydrated in cold temperatures, too.

many cases, athletes choose water or a sports drink and energy gels or portions of uncoated energy bars. (Coatings add saturated fat, which is not something you want in a fast-paced race.) If you're climbing, the type of climbing you're doing affects even how conveniently you'll be able to take a drink. My team in the 1995 Eco-Challenge took a little more than three hours to climb a 1,200-foot cliff using ropes and hardware. On the way up, we periodically drank water and ate bits of bars. A 1,200-foot free climb would be a very different challenge—one that belongs in the final category of "nearly continuous exertion with constrained refueling opportunities."

Nearly Continuous Exertion/Occasional Refueling Opportunities

As mentioned previously, two different types of activities fit into this category: ultra-endurance activities that last more than one day and fast-paced sporting events that last more than an hour.

The latter includes sports like basketball and tennis, in which intense periods of exertion are followed by short breaks that allow you to drink something or maybe down an energy gel. My mother remembers eating orange slices during her basketball games in the 1940s, so the concept of replenishing energy with something light and refreshing isn't new. The delivery systems are just much more efficient now, demanding less of your digestive system. As always, your basic need is water, and hunger isn't necessarily your enemy. If you feel your energy drop, try an energy gel or diluted carb drink to bail you out, but reevaluate your pre-competition program.

For one thing, choose lean sources of protein, rather than red meat, just before the event. Red meat offers some great benefits to athletes, but it's harder to digest than fish and vegetarian sources of protein. Cow's milk and other dairy products are also hard to digest, and they can interfere with the digestion of other nutrients that are important for a race or fast-paced sport. Kevin Maselka, who has trained top professional athletes like basketball star Alonzo Mourning, notes,

> On average, 10 percent of the calories you eat go to digestion. If you take in 1,000 calories, and 10 percent of them are used for digestion, you only have the balance left for the race before you start to deplete your stores, and it becomes a less efficient means of fueling you. Eat efficient types of food.

Surprises invariably await you during a multi-day race. In a foot or cycling race that's always held in the same geographic area, as many of the classic races are—Marathon de Sables, Tour de France, Iterod Extreme, or the Eldoret High Altitude Marathon in Kenya—you can learn from veterans and train for the specific conditions. Adventure races like the Raid Gauloises and Eco-Challenge are everywhere, though, so you have to find out how the indigenous people eat and what the pros eat when they go there.

During the event, no matter what it is, you will want to carry light, nutrient-dense foods. Adventure racer Cathy Sassin's staples for races all over the world include ostrich and turkey jerky, both of which are low-fat protein sources; rollups and bars made solely from fruit; trail mix; nuts; almond paste; and prepackaged, dehydrated foods. Energy bars such as the Canadian Energy to Go (SunRype) and Okanagan Sports Bar

(Okanagan) fit into this plan perfectly. Considering the different kinds of athletic challenges that occur during an adventure race, it is also wise to pack light, uncoated high-calorie bars that will maintain their integrity after being slammed in the bottom of a pack full of climbing hardware. Carry the dehydrated foods in Ziploc plastic bags rather than their original packaging; ultramarathoner Lisa Smith advises adding salt to keep the electrolyte balance in order. If you're in a hot climate, add water to the bag, and then keep going. Your meal will "cook" as you race.

During the event, also give yourself some treats. The psychological boost you get from a fun food can outweigh the nutritional merits of one more energy bar.

Nearly Continuous Exertion/Constrained Refueling Opportunities

In these sports, you can't eat at all while you're competing, and the exertion is steady and intense. The big difference between sports in this category and those in the periodic/occasional category is simply the duration. The most you could hope for is a swig of water.

The important tips for athletes in these sports, therefore, are to build your energy reserves before the event and to be diligent about recovery nutrition. Finally, follow the advice previously given for other athletes in intense-exertion sports: Eat light the day before the event.

Consume Only What You Need

Athletes who must ingest nutrients to get through a competition face different kinds of challenges, depending on whether refueling takes place during a timeout, during a slowdown, or at high speed. During a competition, you want maximum blood flow to go to your muscles, but without a little going to your gut as you take in nutrients, you will get some cramping and potentially other bad effects that will undermine your performance. Help your body function efficiently by eating and drinking only the amounts and types of sports foods you need to stay strong. You will know what those amounts and types are if you keep an accurate log and daily food intake as suggested in chapter 1.

CHAPTER 10

Recharging and Replenishing

Most professional athletes have an off season, a time to recharge and replenish their bodies and spirits through food and training practices they wouldn't use during the competitive season. That doesn't mean they backslide into the land of Krispy Kreme donuts. The more likely scenario is that they try out some different nutritional practices involving whole foods and supplements to see if they can better support on-season athletic goals. Gaining a little weight may be part of the change, but many athletes believe that off-season weight gain is part of a full recovery process.

Regardless of whether you're an elite athlete or an avid amateur, you can benefit from periodically stepping back from your nutritional routine and reevaluating what you ingest as it relates to health and performance. Aging, an increase or decrease in stress, change in a chronic condition, new workout techniques—any of these variables may cause you to investigate some changes. Clinical studies involving sports foods are another reason to revisit what you eat to enhance your athletic performance.

The off season is not necessarily a time of indulgence. It can be a time of cleaning out—eliminating all supplements except those essential for health. Top Ironman triathlete Lori Bowden goes off supplements completely during the off season, when she brings her level of exercise way down. She believes that if she isn't working out hard, she doesn't have a good reason to use them. The off season can also be a period of experimentation, a chance to try out new products or a different approach to diet. Consider the advice of Barry Sears, developer of the Zone diet: "Athletes should always be searching and finding out what's good for their biochemistry. There are no good diets or bad diets, but there is a hormonally correct diet for your biochemistry."

Back to Basics

If you decide to "clean out" to reevaluate how different supplements affect your performance, first think about the hierarchy of these products in your life. Specially formulated foods and supplements can be put into four basic categories in terms of your personal health and fitness needs:

1. Products that alleviate a health problem
2. Products that help you sustain health
3. Products that meet a short-term performance need
4. Products that support your efforts to make a significant physical, performance-related change

This order roughly reflects the hierarchy of their value to your well-being—how much you need them year round.

Supplements for Health

Products that fall into the first category are sometimes referred to as "functional foods," or foods with documented health benefits. The most common types of problems they address for the population at large are obesity, blood cholesterol levels, blood pressure, arteriosclerosis, constipation, osteoporosis, and anemia. If you're a 50-year-old female runner, you'll probably want to take a calcium supplement every day in addition to integrating weight training into your regimen. Many chronic problems that affect athletes, such as Raynaud's disease and the joint pain associated with cartilage deterioration, can be addressed through specially formulated foods and supplements. If you suffer from joint pain and feel relief when you take a glucosamine/chondroitin sulfate supplement, then you probably don't want to drop that from your diet as part of a cleanout program. Similarly, if you lose circulation and feeling in your fingers and toes when they get even slightly cold—the symptoms of Raynaud's disease—then any therapy that helps you should be ongoing. The relief you get by adding essential fatty acids to your diet or taking Heartbar (CookePharma) or Hemo-Flo (Platinum Performance), which are designed to improve circulation, will only be sustained if they are part of a daily program.

Vitamins, minerals, and essential fatty acids (especially omega-3) fall into the category of products that help you sustain health, and so *might* certain herbs, enzymes, amino acids, and other substances. Vitamin E tops the list of supplements you should keep taking during a period of reevaluation, particularly if you're a hard-charging endurance athlete. Some researchers maintain that the amount of vitamin E that endurance athletes need to protect their cells from oxidative damage can't be obtained through food alone. (Among the Web sites with insights and research are the Kansas State University page of references on "Vitamin E and Exercise" and "10 for the Road: Essential Nutrients for Endurance Athletes" listed in the Selected Resources section of this book.

Examples of herbs and enzymes that could have a fundamental role in your health, depending on your age and other circumstances, are digestive enzymes and good bacteria like acidophilus. In general, though, approach the use of herbs with caution and even skepticism, partly because of the questionable purity of some of the products on the market. And keep in mind Barry Sears' warning:

> Herbs consist of alkaloids, and alkaloids are very powerful drugs. Unless you know what you're doing [with them] you can be into some real problems. There is a dose/response effect and at a high enough dose, adverse effects will happen.

Supplements for Performance

The third category of sports foods, those that meet a short-term performance need, encompasses energy and recovery products. As you reassess what works best for you, stop relying on the bars, electrolyte and protein drinks, creatine, and related products for a while. A possible exception is the amino acid glutamine, which you want to continue to take after hard workouts. I've interviewed scores of top athletes about their diets and probed the secrets of success with many strength and conditioning coaches, and the one recovery substance that most of them embrace is glutamine.

A number of whole-food options may deliver results similar to those you get from an energy bar, and you owe it to yourself to try them. It does require more thought and time, however, to tweak your own energy recipe than to buy an off-the-shelf product. The advantage of whole foods is that you can choose to add myriad nutrient-rich, organic fruits and nuts to a basic recipe, thereby adding a lot of variety to your diet. Table 10.1 compares the macronutrient profiles in a few sample snacks and meals that could serve your energy needs. It's intended to give you basic direction in experimenting with your own concoctions.

Keep one thing in mind as you experiment with whole-food alternatives to bars and shakes: The macronutrient profile is not the whole story. The vitamin, mineral, amino acid, and enzyme values of the foods can make a big difference to you as well, and these considerations are explored later in this chapter.

Table 10.1 Macronutrients in Snacks

	Clif Bar (Chocolate Chip Peanut Crunch)	**Odwalla Bar** (Super Protein)	**Trail Mix** (bits of dried fruit, mixed nuts, and seeds)	**Oatmeal** (with raisins)	**Toast** (wheat bran bread, peanut butter, and apple butter)
Serving size	1 bar = 68 gm	1 bar = 62 gm	1/2 cup = 75 gm	1/2 cup oatmeal (40 gm) + 1/4 cup raisins (40 gm) = 80 gm	1 slice bread (36 gm) + 1 tbs. peanut butter (18 gm) + 1 tbs. pure apple butter (19 gm) = 73 gm
Calories	240	230	345	280	280
Carbs (gm)	38	31	34	58	31
Protein (gm)	12	16	11	6	8
Fat (gm) Saturated (gm)	5 1	4 0.5	18 3	3 0.5	7 1
Profile (approx.) carb-protein-fat	63-20-17	55-28-17	40-13-47	82-9-9	45-12-23
Fiber (gm)	5	3	4	6	2

If you make your own trail mix using equal portions of dried fig pieces, dried date pieces, and soy nuts, you'll arrive at a mix with roughly the following characteristics:

70 gram serving:	250 calories
Carbohydrates:	32 grams
Protein:	16 grams
Fat:	7 grams (1.5 saturated)
Macronutrient profile:	approximately 50-26-25

This small amount of mix will also provide you with good amounts of fiber, potassium, calcium, magnesium, and iron. That food value will increase if you carefully select organically grown fruits and nuts. Add a

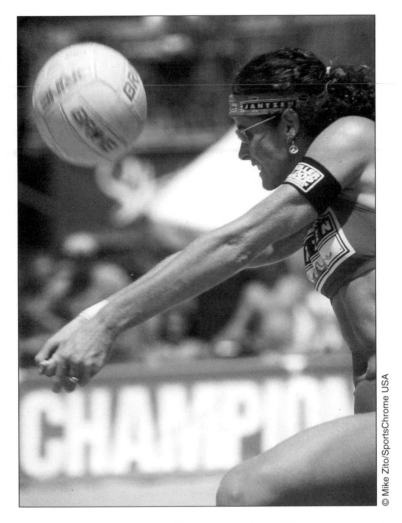

© Mike Zito/SportsChrome USA

You'll perform better on-season if you use the off season to refine your nutritional program.

few almonds, and you'll significantly boost the amount of folic acid, vitamin E, magnesium, and phosphorus in your mix.

Use your off-season exploration to find out how the basic foods affect your energy level. Eat your snack or meal as you would a bar, about an hour before you train. Instead of a protein shake after your weight workout, try eating egg whites that are cooked properly. Never boil eggs; cook them gently over low heat. High heat degrades the protein, which turns the whites into a rubbery mold that has lost much of its value to you. Lower your eggs into simmering water that covers them completely. In three to five minutes, you will have soft-"boiled" eggs; to hard-"boil" them, keep them in the simmering water 12 to 15 minutes.

During this cleanout phase, also try juicing raw vegetables and fruits. The spectrum of nutrients that you can deliver to your body through these juices is amazing. Juicing raw produce takes a lot more time and trouble than dumping a couple of scoops of meal replacement in a blender with water; I don't know more than a few athletes who do this regularly during the competitive season because of the time factor. Treat yourself to it for a while, though, as you try to get down to basics. If you like sweet juices, try a combination of carrot and apple; you can cut the sweetness with lemon juice. If you like an earthy and somewhat sweet taste, juice raw beets, celery, carrots, and a kale leaf. Again, lemon juice will add a tart zing.

During a noncompetitive period, stop using substances in the fourth category—products that support your efforts to make a physical change. This category includes stimulants designed to promote fat loss/muscle gain and prohormones. Avid amateur athletes—nonprofessional sportsmen and women who are more focused on overall fitness than competition—should *always* avoid substances in this category. You have no compelling reason to use products designed to support dramatic physical change such as andro, DHEA, and its relatives in the prohormone category. Your goals and the intensity of your training program are not a good match with these products.

No Supplements, No Extras: The Downs and Ups of Fasting

Some athletes also believe in abstaining from food, water, or both for periods of time to clean out their systems. If you're considering a fast, even one that incorporates fresh juices, then check with your doctor as well as your coach. The merits of any fast depend on the motivation, the duration, and the nature of activity during the fast. Don't fast to lose weight, which has been a common technique of gymnasts and wrestlers through the years. A fast involving dehydration can have particularly devastating implications for very active people. In Clarkson's article (1998), she noted that, in the fall of 1997, "three wrestlers died while performing intense exercise and practicing dehydration procedures." An autopsy report for one of the wrestlers listed rhabdomyolysis as the cause of death. This condition involves a degeneration of muscle cells and is characterized by symptoms such as muscle tenderness, weakness, swelling, brown urine, and increased levels of muscle proteins in the blood. Priscilla, who is associate dean of the school of public health and health sciences at the University of Massachusetts, says that the message in simple terms is this: "Intense exercise in a hot environment can lead to muscle breakdown, which could compromise the kidneys," so taking in fluids is extremely important.

On the other hand, Muslim athletes such as NBA star Hakeem Olajuwon of the Houston Rockets have proven that refraining from food and fluids for an extended period need not degrade athletic performance and may improve an athlete's mental resolve. Their regimen is strict, but it is predictable: The intake of food and water during the fasting period is regular—before dawn and after dusk—and they train their bodies and minds to cope.

Ric Giardina, a devoted amateur cyclist who is a veteran of several AIDS Rides, regularly incorporates fasting into his health and fitness program, and he also does it with spiritual goals in mind:

> Sometimes, my vacations consist of significant amounts of exercise and fasting. Almost every summer I take off for a week or two to the Navaho desert area of the Four Corners area of the southwest. I hike alone into the wilderness and fast (except for vitamins, water, some lemon juice, and about [two to three] tablespoons of honey each day). I'll do that for [three or four] days, then come out, get a hot shower and a light meal, sleep in a bed for a night or two, put the poems I've written while out in the desert into my laptop, and then go out into the wilderness again after a day or two.

Revamping the Diet

Many top athletes have had compelling reasons to use their downtime to reevaluate their diets. Ironman triathletes Lori Bowden and Peter Reid, Olympic gold-medal swimmers Gary Hall Jr. and Dara Torres, and ultra-endurance racer Lisa Smith are just a handful of world-class competitors who had serious issues with what they had been told was a good diet. Gary's challenge, covered in chapter 8, was the most extreme, because he was diagnosed with serious diabetes before the Sydney Olympics in 2000. At critical points in their careers, however, all of the others also felt that the macronutrient profile—that is, the carbohydrate-protein-fat ratio—and the spectrum of micronutrients in their daily diets was not meeting their performance needs.

Peter began his career as a cyclist abiding by the high-carbohydrate, low-protein, low-fat *Eat to Win* diet. But being "the fattest guy on the starting line" didn't give this Canadian champion any performance advantages. He added protein, and he quickly noticed performance results, particularly in the area of recovery. His wife, triathlon champ Lori Bowden, had a similar evolution:

I switched to a balanced diet—it isn't quite 40-30-30—but having more protein and fat in the meal, I find I'm more satisfied with less. It works better than eating a whole pile of carbohydrates calories, and I think my body is burning things more efficiently.

You can see it, too. Instead of having a little definition, you have more muscle definition.

Unlike other athletes, who might casually explore different ways of eating during the off season, gold-medal swimmer Dara Torres had to make a rather abrupt dietary change, and a lot depended on it being the right kind of change. After a seven-year hiatus from elite competition, she lacked the strength and power that coach Richard Quick wanted in members of the U.S. women's swim team, bound for the 2000 Sydney Olympics. She needed more than an ardent desire to become the first American to swim in four Olympics; she needed a lot more muscle. An integral part of her challenge was that Dara did not have a diet that would support big muscle gains:

When I went back into training, I didn't know much about the different kinds of diets. I started doing the Zone. Once I got into it and started to gain muscle—once I got educated about it—it all made sense.

Dara stuck with Barry Sears's Zone diet throughout 13 months of intense training before the Olympics. Her body responded extremely well, and she immediately made progress in gaining lean mass. In about six months, she added 20 pounds of muscle. That's a remarkable gain, even for a 5'11" athlete whose training regimen includes heavy weight workouts. It's even more impressive in light of Dara's focus on diet rather than supplements.

Barry explains that the Zone approach reflects a scientific way of manipulating hormones. It isn't simply a 40-30-30 diet, even though the ratios do apply. If it were a numbers game, then you could get 40 percent of your carbohydrates from white bread, but that's not a food item you find in a Zone diet, which emphasizes vegetables and certain fruits as carb sources. Barry sees Dara's muscle gains and corollary performance improvements as predictable, because of the way the Zone diet aims at triggering hormonal responses:

How can you build better athletes? You want an athlete who has better oxygen transfer. You want an athlete who has better access to stored body fat, a virtually unlimited storehouse of energy. You want an athlete to maintain peak mental awareness, which means that you want stable blood sugar. And you want an athlete who

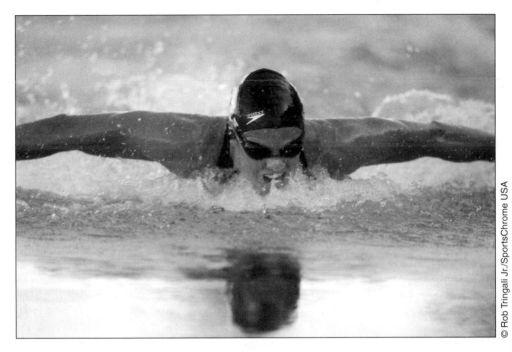

Rob Tringali Jr./SportsChrome USA

Dara Torres revamped her diet with Barry Sears' help and packed on lean muscle.

can maximize the release of growth hormone from the pituitary to repair damaged tissue. Finally, you want to reduce the inflammatory response due to training. All those are under hormonal control and you can achieve that—you can raise your potential closer to your full genetic aspect.

How do you go about maximizing those hormonal responses? There are two primary hormonal responses controlled by the diet (Sears 1995):

1. Insulin, controlled by the ratio of protein to carbohydrates at every meal
2. Eicosanoids, controlled by the ratio of omega-3 to omega-6 fats

Barry's premise with the Zone, therefore, is that consistently eating certain types of carbohydrates, proteins, and fats in the appropriate ratios will give you control over insulin and eicosanoid levels, and hence control over hormonal responses that are key to health and performance. He realizes that requiring people to think a lot in planning meals will not work, however, so he came up with a general guideline to help anyone stay on a Zone-like program:

How [do] you put this in a format that's easy for athletes to follow? All you need is one hand and one eye. This is how you construct meals. No more low-fat protein in one meal than you can fit in the palm in your hand. Take your plate and, at every meal, divide it into three sections. On one third of that plate you put some low-fat protein that's no bigger and thicker than the palm of your hand. On the other two-thirds, fill it with massive piles of fruits and vegetables.

Transforming Sports Foods Into Meals

Convenience is important for busy athletes, which is why Barry's simple explanation is such a great tool in helping them build a Zone-like meal. It is also why meal replacements and protein powders are such attractive options.

Fortunately, a lot of nutrients come along with the convenience of these sports foods. Dump two scoops of powder into a blender of low-fat milk, and voilà, you get 100 percent or more (according to the RDAs) of 12 vitamins and 7 or 8 minerals. In those scoops, however, you may also be getting substances you do not want, such as simple sugars or aspartame to sweeten the powder. Moreover, you probably won't get significant amounts of substances you would get from a balanced meal, such as dietary fiber and healthy fat. In short, a powder-based drink is acceptable if you want to add quality calories, but you have some work to do if you want to transform that product into the foundation of a healthy meal.

Sweeteners: Good, Bad, and Even Politically Incorrect

Read the labels to know what you're consuming.

Aspartame—Aspartame is composed of two amino acids, aspartic acid and phenylalanine, chemically bonded by methanol. People with a genetic disease called phenylketonuria (PKU), which is normally diagnosed by a blood test performed shortly after birth, should avoid aspartame. People with PKU can't properly utilize phenylalanine, so they have to restrict their intake of foods containing this amino acid, such as meat, milk, nuts, and manufactured foods sweetened with aspartame. Some companies, such as Team Pro2 and Hammer Nutrition, completely avoid using aspartame, and others that use it, such as MET-Rx and EAS, clearly mark their labels so that phenylketonurics know to use the products in moderation.

Stevia—A natural noncaloric alternative to artificial sweeteners, stevia has been grown and used safely in South America and Europe for centuries and has been a popular sweetener in Japan for many years, but it is relatively new to the U.S. market. Under the conditions of the Dietary Supplement Health & Education Act, stevia may be used and sold as a food supplement but not a sweetener. (Draw your own conclusions about the artificial sweetener lobby.) As a consequence, manufacturers must be inventive in communicating their use of it as an ingredient. Next Proteins, for example, relies on stevia "for flavor" in its Designer Protein and Isis powders. You may also see stevia marketed as a stand-alone product for therapeutic reasons; it has been used as a digestive aid, an antiseptic, and an antimicrobial substance. Stevia's sweet compounds pass through the digestive process without breaking down, so it should be ideal for athletes, diabetics, hypoglycemics, and anyone else who wants to control their blood-sugar level.

Sugars—Sugars are natural, but that doesn't mean all sugars are equal in terms of your body processes. Even if they have the same name, they don't necessarily share the same characteristics. Chapter 1 presents the basics of sugars, but there are key fine points about sugars that can help you choose among meal-replacement, energy, and recovery products.

First, the phrase "corn syrup" is contained in the names of some sugars with very different characteristics, and "maltodextrin" does not always mean the same thing. Corn syrup refers to a family of sweeteners derived from corn starch. Members of that family include high-fructose corn syrup and maltodextrin. High-fructose corn syrup is an extremely high-glycemic carbohydrate that is used in foods to retain moisture and add a lot of sweetness. It is not an ingredient that you want in sports foods. On the other hand, maltodextrins, which are sometimes labeled glucose polymers, and corn syrup solids can serve athletes well. There is a catch, however. Both of them are often categorized by dextrose equivalence (DE), which is "a measure of the degree of conversion of the starch molecule to the basic glucose molecule" (Singh and Cheryan 1997). This designation gets confusing. Technically speaking, maltodextrin is a carbohydrate with a DE under 20, and glucose syrup (a solution made up mostly of glucose, dextrose, and maltose) is a carbohydrate with a DE above 20, but that doesn't tell you the whole story of either sugar's molecular structure. On one level, you know that the higher the DE, the sweeter the taste

(continued)

and the faster the assimilation, which is why manufacturers who use maltodextrin—a low-DE sugar—promote it as a carbohydrate that delivers long-lasting energy. But the molecular structure of compounds with exactly the same DE can be very different; one may be comprised of lots of long chains and a few short chains (which provide long-lasting energy, but not much of a quick start), while another may have a combination of long chains, medium chains, and short chains.

What that means to you as an athlete is that two different energy gels, meal-replacement products, or other sports foods with maltodextrin can deliver different results. Hammer Nutrition (Hammer Gel), GU, and GOJUS de France are among the manufacturers that emphasize maltodextrins with a greater number of long chains. Formulas can change, however, so you will need to see how you react to the product. Other things you've eaten can also affect how you react, so do your tests in a clean state: hydrated and with a relatively empty stomach.

With a little effort, you can make a meal replacement, protein powder, or certain other kinds of sports foods part of a whole-food experience that gives you a wider spectrum of nutrients. You can also change the macronutrient profile if you like. The following suggestions illustrate ways to accomplish different macronutrient objectives and improve the nutrient values in 275- to 400-calorie meals or snacks involving sports foods. The first three use nonfat yogurt or nonfat milk as an ingredient, but the fourth is a basic nondairy recipe, unless you rely on whey and casein protein products and classify them as dairy products.

Objective: *A small meal with a low amount of dietary fat and a balance of carbohydrates and protein.* Combine nonfat yogurt or nonfat milk with protein powder and add fruit. (The protein powder reflects your personal choice; guidance on the available options is found in chapter 3.) Roughly one cup of yogurt, a 24-gram scoop of powder, one-half cup of strawberries, and one-half banana gives you 275 calories, 37 grams of carbohydrates, 30 grams of protein, and 2 grams of fat, for a profile of 54-44-6.

A meal replacement or protein powder alone will not give you the health and performance benefits associated with the active cultures in quality yogurt and the key nutrients in the fruit. If you use a commercial yogurt, check the label to be sure it contains the good bacterium *lactobacillus acidophilus*, which is what delivers the digestion and antifungal benefits of the product. Fruits such as strawberries and bananas will boost the content of folic acid, which is essential for cell division, tissue growth, and the formation of red blood cells.

A protein powder formulated specifically for women, such as Next Protein's Isis, will already contain a high amount of folic acid, aka folate, (600 mcg). This B vitamin is essential to a healthy pregnancy; the DRI for women who have a chance of getting pregnant is 400 mcg. The powders that most athletes use, however, do not have such a high level of folate.

Strawberries and bananas are two fruits that also boost your dietary potassium, which operates in the fluid inside your cells. As an athlete, you've probably heard many times that cramping can be associated with a potassium deficiency. It can also be associated with sodium and other mineral losses.

These fruits introduce another important factor: fiber. You get almost no dietary fiber by mixing a protein or meal-replacement powder with a dairy product, and even if you combine the powder with juice, you probably get zero fiber. Your body needs fiber to decrease blood lipids and help food move through the GI tract. On the other hand, too much fiber isn't good, either. It can bind with minerals like calcium, iron, and zinc, so that you excrete them instead of absorbing them into your bloodstream. You want about 25 to 30 grams for a 2,000-calorie diet, but if you don't have nearly that much fiber in your diet now, increase the amount slowly to avoid gas, diarrhea, and related GI tract distress. As an athlete, you may be consuming twice that amount of calories, so adjust your fiber intake accordingly. Adding a cup of strawberries or blueberries, one banana, or five tablespoons of raisins to your mixture will put three grams of fiber into your meal. A cup of raspberries will give you three times as much.

When you add a fruit such as strawberries, you also bring a lot of vitamin C to the mixture, as long as you handle the fruit properly. Vitamin C is water soluble, so it leaches out of food as you cook it. It also degrades when it's exposed to light and air. If you want to preserve the vitamin C, cut the fruit immediately before you add it to your mixture. Better yet, don't cut it at all.

Objective: *A small meal with a balance of macronutrients (40-30-30).* Add a tablespoon of flaxseed oil, which provides 13 grams of fat, to the mixture previously described. Flaxseed oil contains linoleic acid and alpha lineolenic acid (ALA), two essential fatty acids that suppress the production of substances that contribute to inflammation in damaged joints. They also support strong immune responses.

Objective: *A small meal that emphasizes carbohydrates but contains a balance of protein and healthy fat.* This breakfast or snack takes no time at all to prepare and is rich in vitamins C and E, fiber, and omega-3 fatty acid. Into a bowl of oat flakes (one and one-quarter cups), pour one cup of nonfat milk and two tablespoons of Platinum Performance food supplement, which is one of the products the U.S. men's swim team relied on in preparation for the Sydney Olympics. The Platinum product, which contains stevia, provides a subtle sweetness. The macronutrient profile of this 300-calorie meal is 50-25-25. You can use a different cereal, such as shredded wheat, to inflate the carbohydrate content, but be cautious in choosing the product. You want grain products that involve only minimal processing.

Objective: *A small nondairy meal that can easily be adjusted to shift the ratios of macronutrients and spectrum of nutrients.* It's amazing what you can do with homemade muesli, protein powder, and juice (or water)—one basic meal can be transformed to offer different tastes, different food values, and different textures. Choose from the following foods:

• Raw whole grains—including rolled oats, oat bran, rye, barley, and wheat bran—offer nutrients such as B vitamins, calcium, potassium, manganese, copper, chromium, selenium, and zinc.

• Dried fruits—like papaya, dates, figs, blueberries, cranberries, and so on—or fresh fruits serve the functions previously described.

• Pumpkin and sunflower seeds and fresh nuts (not roasted) contain many of the same minerals that whole grains offer, but they are also sources of biotin and healthy fats. Biotin is a water-soluble coenzyme that works with B vitamins, helps convert amino acids to protein, and helps metabolize carbohydrates and fatty acids. It is integral to energy production.

• Wheat germ and soy beans are sources of choline, which your body needs to break down fats and reduce lactic acid buildup in muscles.

• Protein powder or meal-replacement powder can regulate the amount of protein and modify the flavor.

• Different juices can add or cut back on sweetness; using water in the mixture is the most neutral option.

An ounce of, say, rolled oats and oat bran combined, will give you 90 calories, with 72 of them coming from 18 grams of carbohydrates. The grains offer some protein, very little fat, and lots of fiber (about four grams). A 24-gram scoop of protein powder also gives you about 90 calories, with 72 of them coming from 18 grams of protein. After combining the grains and protein powder, adjust the mixture by adding fruits, nuts, seeds, and so on, to arrive at the taste and nutrient profile you want on a given day.

Shopping at Green Drugstores

The whole food/sports food combinations suggested above focus on the fact that there is a limit to how much nutrient value you can condense into a designer food product, whether it's a pill or a powder. Until food-making technology takes a giant leap forward into the world of *Star Trek*, you absolutely need the original sources of plant nutrients if you want to enjoy all the benefits of the plants. Another name for plant nutrients, or plant chemicals, is *phytochemicals*. More and more manufacturers are describing phytochemical "solutions" to athletic performance problems in rapturous terms.

They are not necessarily trying to deceive you. They are promoting products based on very early evidence, in some cases, about the role of particular phytochemicals in metabolic processes or health, and based on their confidence that they have been able to bottle the benefits.

The confusion—and hope—lies in the fact that each plant contains hundreds of phytochemicals that contribute to flavor, color, or resistance to disease. Although a reasonable amount is known about phytochemicals with antioxidant properties such as vitamin C, vitamin E, and beta-carotene, many others—bioflavonoids, phenolic substances, chlorogenic and ellagic acids, phytosterols, allicin, and many more—seem to have benefits that may not be captured adequately in supplement form. Until manufacturers learn how to encapsulate the full benefits, eat your fruits, vegetables, legumes, whole grains, seeds, and nuts.

APPENDIX

Sample Comprehensive Health Questionnaire

Medical and nutrition professionals consider these kinds of questions important in helping you customize a program of supplementation. It's a good idea to answer the questions and keep this record in case you seek professional advice. It will also raise your own awareness of conditions that may affect your choice of product or your reaction to it.

Make a note of your history of past illness as well as the habits of your lifestyle.

HISTORY OF PAST ILLNESS		HABITS	
Cancer	❏	Alcoholic beverages	❏
Venereal disease	❏	Tobacco/cigarettes	❏
Congenital abnormalities	❏	Physical inactivity	❏
Other (make a list)	❏	Physical activity (make a list)	❏

Do you currently have or have you had in the past any of the following problems?

GENERAL HEALTH		LOCOMOTOR- MUSCULOSKELETAL	
General weakness	❏	Arthritis	❏
Insomnia	❏	Varicose veins	❏
Stress	❏	Weakness of muscles or joints	❏
Overweight	❏	Any difficulty in walking	❏
Stressful job or life	❏	Recent weight change	❏
Depression	❏	Pain in calves	❏
Tire easily, fatigue	❏	Episodes of muscle or joint pain	❏
Nervousness	❏	Muscle cramps	❏
Appetite loss	❏		

SKIN-NECK

Skin disease ❑

Jaundice ❑

Hives, eczema, or rash ❑

Frequent infection or boils ❑

Abnormal pigmentation,
  change in mole ❑

Acne ❑

Stiffness or change in
  size of neck ❑

Enlarged glands in neck ❑

HEAD-EARS-EYES-NOSE-THROAT

Head injury concussion ❑

Lightheadedness ❑

Spots or shades before
  your eyes ❑

Eye disease or injury ❑

Do you wear glasses ❑

Double vision or visual
  disturbances ❑

Impaired hearing,
  hearing change ❑

GASTROINTESTINAL

Peptic ulcer
  (stomach or duodenal) ❑

Vomiting blood or food ❑

Gallbladder disease ❑

Recent change in bowel
  movements ❑

Hepatitis ❑

Painful bowel movements ❑

Bleeding with bowel
  movements ❑

Cramping or pain in the
  abdomen ❑

RESPIRATORY

Frequent head colds ❑

Spitting up blood ❑

Chronic or frequent cough ❑

Asthma or wheezing ❑

Difficulty or shortness
  of breath ❑

Any trouble with lungs ❑

Pleurisy or pneumonia ❑

Tuberculosis ❑

Exposed to dust, fumes ❑

Itching eyes or nose ❑

Sneezing or runny nose ❑

Nosebleeds ❑

Chronic sinus trouble ❑

Ear disease or ringing
  in the ear ❑

Exposure to loud noise ❑

Glaucoma ❑

Dizziness or transient
  blackouts ❑

Heartburn or indigestion ❑

Hemorrhoids ❑

Liver trouble ❑

Constipation ❑

Frequent diarrhea ❑

Excess gas ❑

Black stools ❑

Sigmoidoscopy of the colon ❑

Does food ever stick in the
  throat? ❑

Even minor experiences with these can be very significant if you are considering any of the fat burners, as well as some of the other products with prohormones or herbs.

CARDIOVASCULAR

Stroke ❏

Heart attack ❏

Rheumatic fever or
   heart disease ❏

Chest pain, tight chest,
   or angina ❏

Shortness of breath,
   walking or lying ❏

Difficulty walking one
   or two blocks ❏

Heart trouble or
   heart attacks ❏

Arrhythmia ❏

Thrombophebitis ❏

High blood pressure ❏

Swelling of the hands,
   feet, or ankles ❏

Awakening in the night,
   smothering ❏

Occasional irregular heart
   beats ❏

Heart palpitates,
   beats too hard, flutters ❏

Aware of pulsations
   in the abdomen ❏

High cholesterol or
   triglycerides ❏

Abnormal circulation test,
   examination ❏

Heart murmur or mitral
   valve prolapse ❏

Leg cramps at rest or at night ❏

Coldness of hands or feet ❏

Color changes in toes or feet ❏

Discoloration, ulcers,
   sores of leg or feet ❏

GENITURINARY

Diabetes ❏

Constantly thirsty ❏

Loss of urine ❏

Frequent urination ❏

Change in urinary habit ❏

Night-time urination ❏

Burning or painful
   urination ❏

Blood in urine ❏

Kidney trouble ❏

Kidney stones ❏

Water retention ❏

NEUROLOGICAL

Backpains/problems ❏

Fainting spells—ever ❏

Convulsions or tremors ❏

Paralysis ❏

Numbness, tingling of arm,
   leg, or face ❏

Weakness of arm, leg,
   or facial muscle ❏

Twitching of muscles ❏

Memory problems ❏

Loss of coordination ❏

ENDOCRINE

Allergies ❏

Thyroid disease or
medication ❏

Change in tolerance to
heat or cold ❏

Ever taken any steroids
for any reason ❏

HEMATOLOGIC

Cuts or bruises slow
to heal ❏

Any blood disease

Anemia, past or present ❏

Phlebitis or thrombosis ❏

Abnormal bleeding of
any kind ❏

GYNECOLOGICAL

Any pain with periods ❏

Change in regularity
of periods ❏

Ever had a mammogram ❏

Ever use birth control pills ❏

Date of last pap smear ❏

Results of previous
pap smears ❏

OPERATIONS

Make a list of all your
surgeries ❏

You should also take a look at your family history. Scan your answers and see if you spot any patterns that could signal a problem you may encounter later. For example, if you have never had the slightest indication of a heart problem, but members of your family have experienced heart trouble, you may want to consult a doctor before you take products with a lot of stimulants. And if you have several cases of cancer in your family, you may somehow be predisposed to a cancerous condition. Taking prohormones could put you at great risk.

For the same reason, make a list of any medications you currently take, including vitamins and minerals.

You want to have a complete record of what you were doing and how you felt before embarking on a new program so you have a clear understanding of how the performance-enhancing products affect you.

GLOSSARY

adenosine triphosphate (ATP)—The body's direct energy supply; a chemical substance required for all muscular activity. ATP results when food and oxygen are combined. (The other products are carbon dioxide and water.)

amino acids—The building blocks of protein. The sequence of the amino acids in a protein determines what job it will have in body processes.

anabolic—Muscle building.

Androstenediol—A prohormone, or testosterone precursor, in the same family as Androstenedione. (See *Androstenedione.)*

Androstenedione—A hormone precursor of testosterone, or pro-hormone.

aromatization—A natural process that converts testosterone to estrogen.

Beta-hydroxy beta-methylbutyrate monohydrate (HMB)—Occurs naturally but supplementation used as a possible way of preventing muscle breakdown.

biological value (BV)—A measure of the quality of protein.

blood glucose—Blood sugar.

branched chain amino acids (BCAAs)—Leucine, isoleucine and valine; needed during exercise to maintain muscle tissue, sustain the muscle glycogen supply, and help prevent muscle breakdown.

carbohydrate—A ready source of fuel for both the body and the brain; breaks down into glucose. Composed of carbon, hydrogen, and oxygen.

carbohydrate loading—A technique to boost muscle glycogen stores in advance of a long endurance event; classic approach involves a six-day regimen that goes from low to very high carbohydrate intake.

casein—A protein found in milk that forms curds when exposed to acid and is difficult for infants to digest.

catabolism—Breakdown of muscle tissue.

chelation—The process of bonding a mineral to an amino acid to make the supplement easier to digest and assimilate.

chondroitin sulfate—A naturally occurring substance in the body that slows joint deterioration and reduces the joint pain associated with injury and cartilage degeneration.

chrysin—A substance that minimizes the conversion of testosterone to estrogen.

complete protein—Protein that has all the essential amino acids.

complex carbohydrates—Combinations of the simple sugars.

cortisol (aka *hydrocortisone*)—A hormone of the adrenal gland; linked with a catabolic effect.

creatine loading—A one-week program of high dosages of creatine, which theoretically boosts the body's store of creatine phosphate.

creatine phosphate—An amino acid the body breaks down at moments of peak output to resupply ATP to the muscles.

dehydroepiandrosterone (DHEA)—A hormone precursor of testosterone.

Dietary Reference Intakes (DRIs)—The latest revision of the Recommended Daily Allowances (RDAs).

diuretic—A substance that causes the body to release water.

electrolytes—Sodium, potassium, calcium, magnesium, and chloride.

ephedra—The herbal form of ephedrine, used for years to counter obesity in adults.

essential fatty acids (EFAs)—"Good" fats needed for strong cell walls, metabolism, and other important functions.

fat—Needed to metabolize the fat-soluble vitamins A, D, E, and K; rich source of stored energy. Composed of carbon, hydrogen, and oxygen.

flaxseed oil—Contains linoleic acid and alpha lineolenic acid (ALA), both of which are essential fatty acids.

Food Circle—The author's graphic depiction of how athletes need to build a balanced diet; the greatest area is devoted to water.

Food Pyramid—The United States Department of Agriculture's graphic depiction of the ideal number of servings of each type of food; not a good guide for building an athlete's diet. (See *Food Circle.*)

fructose—The main type of sugar in fruit; often used by diabetics as a sweetener.

glucosamine—A substance that occurs naturally in the body and helps to keep cartilage spongy.

glucose—The main sugar in blood, which serves as the basic body fuel.

glutamine—An amino acid that is key to recovery.

glycemic index (GI)—A guide that rates foods according to how fast they raise blood sugar levels.

glycerol (aka *glycerin, glycerine,* and *glycerate*)—A liquid used in medicines and cosmetics; often used in protein bars to add moisture. Estimated calorie value is four calories per gram.

glycogen—Glucose stored in the muscles and liver.

HMB—See *beta-hydroxy beta-methylbutyrate monohydrate.*

human growth hormone (HGH)—A hormone produced and secreted by the pituitary gland; converted in the liver to insulin growth factor 1. (See *insulin growth factor 1.*)

hydrolyzed protein—Protein that has been bathed to break down amino acids.

hypoglycemia—Low blood sugar.

hyponeutremia—A potentially fatal imbalance involving too much water and not enough sodium in the body.

insulin—A hormone released after eating, which the body needs to process foods properly.

insulin growth factor 1 (IGF-1)—Belongs to a family of proteins that is important for normal human growth and development.

ketogenic diet—A low-carbohydrate program, such as Atkins Diet.

ketosis—Increased blood acids; a potentially dangerous side effect of carbohydrate depletion.

L-carnitine – Often mislabeled an amino acid, but actually more like a vitamin; the body makes it out of lysine and methionine, which are amino acids.

lactic acid system—One of the two anaerobic (without oxygen) energy systems. (See *phosphocreatine system.)*

macronutrient—The macronutrients are carbohydrates, protein, and fat.

maltodextrin—A complex carbohydrate that is easily absorbed.

medium chain triglycerides (MCTs)—A type of saturated fat often found in ketogenic (low-carbohydrate) diets.

melatonin—A hormone associated with restful sleep.

muscle glycogen— Sugar stored in the muscle.

nandrolone (aka *nortestosterone*)—A hormone that remains attached to steroid receptors longer than testosterone.

net protein utilization (NPU)—A measure of the quality of protein.

nonsteroidal anti-inflammatory drug (NSAID)—A drug that subdues the pain related to joint damage; examples are naproxen, ibuprofen, and aspirin.

Norandrostenedione—A prohormone that is converted not to testosterone but to nandrolone. (See *nandrolone.)*

phosphocreatine system—One of the two anaerobic (without oxygen) energy systems. (See *lactic acid system.)*

phytochemicals—Plant nutrients, or plant chemicals.

prohormone—A hormone precursor of testosterone.

protein—A substance needed for muscle growth and repair, the formation of new tissues, and fighting diseases; antibodies and other elements of the immune system are proteins. Consists of amino acids composed of carbon, hydrogen, oxygen, nitrogen, and sulfur.

protein efficiency ratio (PER)—A measure of the quality of protein.

Recommended Dietary Allowances (RDAs)—A description of adequate quantities of key nutrients for normal, healthy people under usual environmental stresses; developed by the Food and Nutrition Board of the National Academy of Sciences.

ribose—A sugar that forms the base of ATP. (See *adenosine triphosphate.)*

saturated fat—"Bad" fat found in meat and dairy products and in certain plant oils, such as coconut and palm. Generally, the more liquid a fat is at room temperature, the less saturated it is.

simple sugars—Glucose, fructose, and galactose.

taurine—An amino acid.

thermogenic aid—A diet aid; that is, a fat-burning agent.

trace minerals (aka *trace elements*)—Important for health. Daily minimums exist for four (iron, zinc, iodine, and selenium), and "safe and adequate" daily ranges have been set for five others (copper, manganese, fluoride, chromium, and molybdenum). The body needs at least five other trace minerals, but research on useful dosages is ongoing.

tribulus terrestris—An herb that some European studies have linked with elevation of testosterone levels.

whey—Proteins, such as lactalbumin, that are found in great amounts in human milk and are easy to digest.

ZMA—Zinc aspartate and magnesium aspartate; taken at night to promote anabolic effects.

SELECTED RESOURCES

Anthony, J.C., T.A. Gautsch, and D.K. Layman. 1999. Leucine supplementation enhances skeletal muscle recovery in rats following exercise. *Journal of Nutrition* 129: 1102-1106.

Baylor College of Medicine: **www.bcm.tmc.edu**

Christianson, A. 1999. 10 for the road: essential nutrients for endurance athletes. *Nutrition Science News* (May). Accessible at **www.healthwellexchange.com**

Gautsch, T.A., J.C. Anthony, S.R. Kimball, G.L. Paul, D.K. Layman, and L.S. Jefferson. 1998. Availability of eIF4E regulates skeletal muscle protein synthesis during recovery from exercise. *American Journal of Physiology: Cell Physiology* 274(2): C406-C414.

Gautsch, T.A., S.M. Kandl, S.M. Donovan, and D.K. Layman. 1999. Growth hormone promotes somatic and skeletal muscle growth recovery in rats following chronic protein-energy malnutrition. *Journal of Nutrition* 129: 828-837.

Kansas State University page of references on *Vitamin E and Exercise:* fn635/vite/ref.htm" **www.oznet.ksu.edu/ed_fn635/vite/ref.htm**

Layman, D.K., R. Boileau, J. Painter, D. Erickson, H. Shiue, and C. Sather. 2000. Carbohydrates versus protein in diets for mid-life women. *FASEB Journal* 14: A564.

Layman, D.K., and G. Wisont. 1999. Leucine stimulates clearance of indispensable amino acids. *FASEB Journal* 13: A908.

Paul, G.L., T.A. Gautsch, and D.K. Layman. 1997. Amino acid and protein metabolism during exercise and recovery. In *Nutrition in exercise and sport, 3rd ed.*, ed. I. Wolinsky, 125-158. Boca Raton: CRC Press.

The Physician and Sportsmedicine Online web site: **www.physsportsmed.com/issues/sailing/sailing.htm**

Shiue, H., C. Sather, and D.K. Layman. 2001. Reduced carbohydrate/protein ratio enhances metabolic changes associated with weight loss diet. *FASEB Journal.* 15: A301.

REFERENCES

Bloomstrand E., P. Hassmen, and B. Ekblom. 1991. Administration of branch-chain amino acids during sustained exercise - effects on performance and on plasma concentration of some amino acids. *European Journal of Applied Physiology* 63: 83-8.

Boirie, Y., M. Dangin, P. Gachon, M.P. Vasson, J.L. Maubois, and B. Beaufrere. 1997. Slow and Fast Dietary Proteins Differently Modulate Postprandial Protein Accretion. *Proceedings of the National Academy of Sciences* 94: 14930-35. Accessible at: **http://www.pnas.org**.

Brooks, G.A., and T.D. Fahey. 1984. *Exercise physiology: human bioenergetics and its applications.* New York: John Wiley and Sons.

Brouns F., J.A. Hawley, and A.E. Jeukendrup. 1998. The effect of rehydration drinks on post-exercise electrolyte excretion in trained athletes. *International Journal of Sports Medicine* 19(1)(January): 56-60.

Castell L.M., J.R. Poortmans, and E.A. Newsholme. 1996. Does glutamine have a role in reducing infections in athletes? *Eur. J. Appl. Physiology* 73(5): 488-90.

Clarkson, P. M. 1998. Exertional rhabdomyolysis. *The NCAA News, Sports Sciences Newsletter* (October 26).

Dorfman, L. 2000. *The vegetarian sports nutrition guide.* New York: John Wiley and Sons.

Furchgott, R., F. Murad, and L. Ignarro, 1998 Nobel Prize/Medicine winning research uncovered the role nitric oxide plays in fighting heart disease.

Garlick P. J., and I. Grant. 1988. Amino acid infusion increases the sensitivity of muscle protein synthesis in vivo to insulin. *Biochem. J.* 254: 579-584.

Gershoff, S. 1996. *The Tufts University guide to total nutrition.* New York: Harper.

Lai, E.C., K. Felice, B.W. Festoff, et al. 1995. A double-blind, placebo-controlled study of recombinant human insulin-like growth factor I in the treatment of amyotrophic lateral sclerosis. *Ann. Neurol.* 38: 971.

Lappe, M. 1976. *Diet for a small planet.* New York: Ballantine Books.

Maughan, R.J., and S.M. Shirreffs. 1998. Fluid and electrolyte loss and replacement in exercise. In Harries, M., C. Williams, W.D. Stanish, and L.L. Micheli, 97-113. *Oxford textbook of sports medicine, 2nd ed.* New York: Oxford University Press.

Misner, B. 2000. Muscle recovery from extreme endurance events: Assessing the damages... The "awful afters"—Counting the cost of a 140-mile trans-sahara footrace. E-Caps and Hammer Nutrition. Posted by the American Fitness Professionals and Associates at **www.afpafitness.com/articles/MuscleRecovery.htm.**

NCAA. 2000. Legislative assistance, NCAA Bylaw 16.5.2.2 (Proposal No. 99-72). *The NCAA News* (August 20).

Rodriguez R., 1998. Medical dispatches from the Whitbread sailboat race. *The Physician and Sportsmedicine Online.* March 18. Accessible at: **www.physsportsmed.com/issues/sailing/sailing.htm.**

Rohde T., D.A. Maclean, and B.K. Pedersen. 1998. Effect of glutamine supplementation on changes in the immune system induced by repeated exercise. *Med. Sci. Sports Exercise* (June): 30(6): 856-862.

Sakurada, B., D. Pharm, and J. Carnazzo. 1999. RPh Effervescent creatine: Facts and fallacies. *FSI Nutrition.* **www.fsinu.com/studies/facts.htm.**

Sears, Barry. 1995. *Enter The Zone.* New York: Harper Collins.

Singh, A., and B. Day. 1989. Magnesium, zinc and copper status of 270 U.S. Navy Sea, Air and Land (SEAL) Trainees. *American Journal of Clinical Nutrition* 49 (April): 695–700.

Singh, N., and M. Cheryan. 1997. Microfiltration for clarification of corn starch hydrolysates. *Cereal Foods World* 42(1) (1997): 21–24.

Stout, J.R., J.M. Eckerson, K. Ebersole, G. Moore, S. Perry, T. Housh, A. Bull, J. Cramer, and A. Batheja. 2000. The effect of creatine loading on the neuromuscular fatigue threshold. *Journal of Applied Physiology.* 88: 109-112.

Stryer, Lubert. 1995. *Biochemistry, 4th ed.* New York: W.H. Freeman and Co.

Sullivan P.G., J.D. Geiger, M.P. Mattson, and S.W. Scheff. 2000. Dietary supplement creatine protects against traumatic brain injury. *Ann. Neurol.* 48 (November): 723-729.

Vandenberghe, K., N. Gillis, M. Van Leemputte, P. Van Hecke, F. Vanstapel, and P. Hespel. 1996. Caffeine counteracts the ergogenic action of muscle creatine loading. *Journal of Applied Physiology* 80: 452–457.

Wardlaw, G.W. 2000. Glossary. Medical terminology to aid in the study of nutrition. *Contemporary Nutrition: Issues and Insights, 4th Ed.* Boston: McGraw Hill.

Zvosec, D.L., and S.W. Smith. 2000. GHB, GBL and 1,4-butanediol intoxication. *The Poison Line: The Newsletter of the American Association of Poison Control Centers* 19(1): (February).

INDEX

Note: The italicized *f* and *t* following page numbers refer to figures and tables, respectively.

ABOUT THE AUTHOR

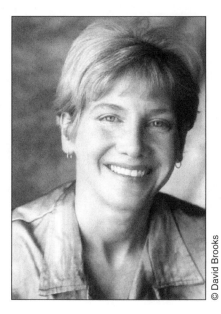

© David Brooks

Maryann Karinch has written numerous books and articles on fitness and nutrition, including *Lessons from the Edge,* a book featuring stories and how-to insights from athletes in extreme sports; and *Boot Camp,* a humorous back-to-basics fitness plan, coauthored by Patrick "The Sarge" Avon.

An avid competitor in endurance and outdoor sports, Karinch began her serious study of nutrition in an effort to improve her own performance without the use of anabolic steroids. She has successfully competed in power lifting and National Physique Committee bodybuilding events, and she was a member of one of the few teams to complete the inaugural Eco-Challenge in southern Utah. She was also a collegiate regional gymnastics champion.

Karinch has continued her advanced nutrition studies as a certified personal trainer with the American Council on Exercise (ACE). She holds an MA in speech and drama from the Catholic University of America and lives in Half Moon Bay, California, where she enjoys ocean whitewater kayaking, weight training, and cooking.